The Enduring Human Spirit

Thought-Provoking Stories on Caring for Our Elders

Including Challenging "Questions for Reflection"

Charles Tindell

Idyll Arbor
Ravensdale, WA

Idyll Arbor, Inc.

PO Box 720, Ravensdale, WA 98051 (425) 432-3231

Idyll Arbor, Inc. Editors: Beverley H. Burlingame and Thomas M. Blaschko

To the best of our knowledge, the information and recommendations of this book reflect currently accepted practice. Nevertheless, they cannot be considered absolute and universal. Recommendations for a particular client must be considered in light of the client's needs and condition. The author and publisher disclaim responsibility for any adverse effects resulting directly or indirectly from the suggested practices, from any undetected errors, or from the reader's misunderstanding of the text.

ISBN 1-882883-51-9

Library of Congress Cataloging-in-Publication Data

Tindell, Charles.
  The enduring human spirit : thought-provoking stories on caring for our elders : including challenging "questions for reflection" / Charles E. Tindell.
    p. ; cm.
  ISBN 1-882883-51-9 (pbk. : alk. paper)
  1. Aged--Case studies. 2. Nursing home patients--Case studies. 3. Quality of life--Case studies. I. Title.
  HQ1061.T497 2003
  305.26--dc21

                                                                        2003007561

Dedicated to:

My wife, Carol

My son, Scott, his wife, Jennifer,
and his children, Julia and Alexander

My son, Andrew, his wife, Lisa,
and his children, Benjamin and Joshua

My son, Robert.

Contents

A friend is better than a thousand silver pieces.
— Greek Proverb

All wisdom is not taught in your school.
— Hawaiian Proverb

Every path has a puddle.
— English Proverb

Love has no law.
— Portuguese Proverb

Who gives to me, teaches me to give.

— Dutch Proverb

Character is a line on stone; none can rub it out.

— African Proverb

Heroism consists in hanging on one minute longer.

— Norwegian Proverb

Heaven has many cracks through which God can see.

— Russian Proverb

> ***Old age, to the unlearned, is winter; to the learned, it is harvest time.***
>
> — Yiddish Proverb

If you wish to know the road ahead, inquire of those who have traveled it.

— *Chinese Proverb*

Preface

According to the dictionary, a proverb is "a brief popular epigram or maxim." The reason I chose to use them throughout this book is that they also can represent the collective wisdom gathered from the life experiences of those who have traveled the journey before us.

The stories within this book are of individuals whose lives are testimonies to the ageless human spirit. As in my previous book, *Seeing Beyond the Wrinkles*, these stories come from men and women who reside in a nursing home.

I am sure many of you have your own *proverbs of life* that you have learned from parents, grandparents, relatives, or friends who have already finished or are now on that last part of their pilgrimage in life. Their stories give insights into what it means to meet the challenges of life with courage, faith, wit, and humor. Their wisdom and values are their gifts to us. The stories we share with each other may be considered gifts and they become legacies to future generations. The stories of the men and women in this book are also legacies that we can benefit from and learn from; the stories are their gifts to us.

Harold (Always Aim for the Bull's-eye), in his eighties and confined to a wheelchair, lived and taught by example his belief that one should shoot for the bull's-eye. What he meant was that we should live each day to its fullest; that we should never, regardless of age or circumstance, short-change ourselves in experiencing life. He tried to give each day what he called his "best shot." When he died, he left that philosophy as a legacy for all to embrace.

Lester (A Darn Good Storyteller) was a most unique individual. At the time of his death, at the age of ninety-four, he no longer had any living relatives, and he had outlived most of his friends. The staff and other residents had become his surrogate family. His legacy comes from a question he scrawled on a scrap of paper and gave to a nurse years ago. The nurse now has the note tacked to the bulletin board above her desk, and it serves as a reminder of the reasons she is devoting her life's work to providing care for the elderly. Lester's question was "Do you ever visit the old and sick?" If we hear his question as only a haunting cry from a lonely old man, we negate something of Lester, and we lose the opportunity to hear a call to reflect upon and rediscover what all of us share in common as human beings. His question calls us to reflect upon what it means to care for one another as we journey the pathway through life.

Zelma (My Friend Flicka) is an individual who epitomizes the enduring, ageless human spirit. With a positive attitude and a sense of humor, she meets the problems that come with the aging process. While being realistic about what lay ahead, nevertheless, her enthusiasm for living life to the fullest each day is a role model for young and old alike.

The above three individuals (and all the others in this book) encourage us to always aim for the bull's-eye while reminding us that the basic values of life have no age boundaries.

All the stories you are about to read are based on real people. To respect and protect the privacy of the individuals involved, names and certain particulars of their stories have been changed. While the individuals described are those who live in a nursing home and are sometimes referred to as the "frail elderly," their courage, strength, and ageless spirits are anything but frail. How they deal with the challenging circumstances within their lives will be appreciated by persons of any age as their stories remind us of what is important in life.

The following pages are filled with truly remarkable individuals, some of whose stories you may want to pin on *your* bulletin board, and whose legacies you may wish to embrace.

Note: At the end of each section, there are **Questions for Reflection**. These questions are designed to help all of us who are interested in the elderly (whether we are elderly ourselves or are caretakers, family members, and friends) when considering the important questions of how we want to treat our elders. By asking the questions, we can think about the tough issues involved in maintaining dignity and human rights at the ends of our lives in long-term care, home health care, and other end-of-life situations.

You may wish, as a token of your appreciation, to provide a copy of this book to those who have the responsibility of caring for your loved one.

Everyone is the age of their heart.

— *Guatemalan Proverb*

Introduction

Who Will Benefit From This Book and How?

The elderly will benefit. They will be affirmed as human beings whose courage, faith, wit, and humor are an inspiration to all ages. They also will be encouraged as they read about Clarence, Elizabeth, Claire, and others, and how they and their peers are dealing with all the challenges life brings in that final phase of one's journey in life. They will be pleased to have a book to give to their family and friends that speaks for them and their circumstances. They will be able to say, *Read this and understand.*

Those in their 50's and 60's will benefit. They will gain insights about the aging process as it affects their parents, other relatives, and friends. Through stories such as those about Margaret, Sid, and Lyle, they will see that although the *Golden Years of Retirement* may be a little tarnished, those years cannot tarnish the power of the human spirit. They will be pleased to see the variety of ways in which older people still give of themselves regardless of age or circumstances. In all of this, they will discover positive role modeling for aging being set forth by their elders.

Those in their 30's and 40's will benefit. They will gain a better understanding of the physical, emotional, mental, and spiritual challenges their parents and others of that generation face in approaching the retirement years. Through the stories of Audrey, Virgil, Stan, and others, they will see that although wheelchairs and walkers are symbols of a weakening physical condition, they are not necessarily signs of a weakening human spirit. From these people they will learn that the values of yesterday are still valid today.

Teens and young adults will benefit. The stories of Zelma, Herman, Daisy, and Leo, for example, will ask them to see beyond the wrinkles and to peer into the youthful hearts of the elderly. They will understand that they and the elderly share the same need for such things as independence, dignity, and respect. In addition, they will find themselves on common ground with the elderly as those of both generations battle assumptions based on stereotypical images people have of them, whether those assumptions concern young people on skateboards or elderly in wheelchairs. After reading these stories, they will have a better appreciation of the challenges facing their grandparents and great-grandparents and of the positive ways their elders are coping with whatever the years may bring.

All **staff (dietary, housekeeping, activities, administration, social services, nursing, etc.) of long-term care facilities or retirement communities will benefit.** At the end of each selection of stories, there is a section entitled *Questions for Reflection.* The questions are designed to encourage, as well as challenge, staff to look at their work differently. How people have been cared for in the past cannot be assumed to be the model for how they are cared for now or in the future. These sections are meant to be a catalyst for discussion. They can be useful for staff training, new staff orientation, team meetings, etc.

Who hears but one bell hears but one sound.

— French Proverb

The Wizard of Oz

A tornado warning had just been issued over the radio and eighty-eight-year-old Herman was ecstatic.

Sirens in the distance could be heard sounding the alarm in adjacent communities. Our facility had taken action according to its Severe Weather Emergency Plan: residents' window shades had been pulled down and the curtains drawn to reduce the risk of injury by flying glass; those residents who could be moved were moved into the corridors; all residents were being accounted for in each area by a head count; staff were at assigned locations. Everything was going according to procedure — that is, almost everything. The one exception was Herman who was relaxing in his wheelchair, gazing up into the threatening sky and studying the turbulent clouds. He was in front of the building, "parked" at the end of the sidewalk. Herman had never seen a tornado and was determined to have that experience before he reached his approaching eighty-ninth birthday.

Other staff asked me to see if I, as the chaplain, could convince Herman to come inside the building. I said I'd try, but I knew that Herman could be hardheaded and ornerier than a jackass. That isn't my description but rather his own, and he was quite proud of it.

"This place needs a stubborn SOB just to add some color and character," he would say in a voice that sounded like a truck rolling slowly down a gravel road. "It's too dull around here. Don't you think so?"

Herman could be a cantankerous old cuss to be sure, but a lovable one. One staff member had said of him, "One minute he'd get me so angry I could scream, and the very next minute he'd charm the socks right off me with his grin and the way he winked when he was doing something he knew he wasn't supposed to be doing. How can he can be so infuriating and charming at the same time?"

As I walked out to where Herman was, I noted that he had his pipe in his mouth. I thought to myself, *He's up to his old tricks again.* Our facility recently adopted a policy declaring it a non-smoking facility. Those few residents who smoked at the time when the policy went into effect were grandfathered in as the last of the residents who would be allowed to smoke. Herman was one of them. He and the others, however, were permitted to smoke only in a designated area. All other areas, including the outside grounds, were off limits. Herman displayed his disapproval of the policy by always having his pipe with him, and in his mouth whenever he figured staff would cross paths with him. Seeing the pipe in his mouth, a staff person would remind him that smoking was allowed only in the designated area. The trap set, Herman would curtly reply, "Do you see any smoke coming from this pipe?"

"Well, no, I don't."

"Ain't lit, is it?"

"No."

"Any policy preventing me from having an unlit pipe in my mouth?"

"No."

"Damn right there isn't," he would exclaim triumphantly. "Leave me alone then and go bother some other poor resident."

There have been occasions when I've come upon Herman in a non-smoking area and could smell the burnt tobacco and see white ashes in the bowl of his pipe. "How're you doing?" I would ask as I glanced at his pipe so Herman would know that I knew what he was up to.

"Doing okay, Boss," he would reply (for some reason, he always called me Boss) and then he would wink at me as he tapped the bowl of the pipe against his pant leg with one hand while reaching for his tobacco pouch with the other.

Herman, a self-made man, often shared stories of his parents and the struggles they had coming to America from their native land of Latvia. He was proud of his family's history and their European roots, but he also took a special pride in this country to which his parents had emigrated and in which he had been born. For Herman, ideals such as freedom and independence were not meant to be celebrated only during one or two holidays a year. His parents had taught him to treasure these values, and he considered them so important that he tried to live them every day of his life. They became even more meaningful to Herman as he carried them with him into his later years of life. Confinement to a wheelchair wouldn't stop him from exercising what he considered to be his God-given rights. Herman was convinced that somewhere in the Constitution of the United States of America there were certain inalienable rights about old men who wanted to smoke their pipes and celebrate their birthdays in any damn way they pleased.

Approaching him that day, the sirens screaming and the clouds tumbling above us, his first words were, "Boss, you ain't going to tell me I have to come in like all those others have, are you?"

"No," I replied, quickly reconsidering how I should handle the situation. "I'm just wondering what you're out here for." I surveyed the threatening sky. "It looks like pretty stormy weather to me," I said, hoping that he would get the message.

"Lived in Minnesota damn near all my life," he growled. "Never have seen one of those tornadoes they're always talking about. Thought maybe I'll get to see one today." Looking up at the clouds swirling about, Herman scratched the back of his head with his pipe stem as he added, "Hell, I don't think so, though. Some pretty clouds up there; don't you think?"

Visions of Herman being swept up by a tornado, whisked off in his wheelchair like Dorothy in the Wizard of Oz, went through my mind. As we talked, a staff person who had been checking the outside grounds for any other residents walked toward us. Herman turned toward me and growled, "Five." I didn't realize what he meant until the staff person began to inform him that he should come indoors. Before she got halfway through, he interrupted, pointed the stem of his pipe toward her, and said with a scowl, "You're the fifth person who's told me to come in. I'll come in when I'm damn good and ready."

The staff person looked at me and then back at Herman, shrugged her shoulders and said in a voice brimming with frustration, "Okay, but we're going to document this, and if anything happens to ..."

"Go ahead and document it," Herman roared. "I don't give a damn."

Exasperated, she stormed away as still another staff person came walking toward us. "Six," Herman said calmly as he filled his pipe with fresh tobacco. After dismissing number six, he resumed his inspection of the darkening clouds, his eyes squinting. "No, Boss," he said to me, "I don't think I'll see myself one of those tornadoes today. What do you think?"

"I think you might be right," I replied, hoping he wouldn't catch the uncertainty in my voice. He didn't know how hard I was praying that he was right. "I tell you what," I offered. "I'll stay out here until it begins to rain and then we'll go in. What do you say to that? Is it a deal?"

"Oh, oh, here comes number seven," he said, winking at me.

Some time later Herman finally did go in, but only after it began to rain quite hard and the wind picked up. As he let me wheel him back into the safety of the building, he chuckled and said in his raspy voice, "Well, Boss, how did we do? Ten or eleven?"

"Ten," I replied, not being able to suppress a smile.

Herman died several months later. At his Service of Remembrance most of those ten staff people were there sharing stories about this stubborn, contentious man who so deeply touched their hearts.

Ghosts and Spirits, But No Goblins

There are *ghosts* (or *spirits*, if you prefer) who roam our facility. One is that of Palmer, a former resident, who died six years ago. The other ghost (or spirit) is that of Dottie, a nurse who worked at the nursing home and then, in her later years, lived there as a resident. She died over twenty years ago. Without rattling chains or appearing as apparitions, Dottie and Palmer still find ways to make their presence felt. Their legends continue to grow with each passing year. First, let me tell you about Palmer.

Palmer was a resident for nearly seven years, all of which were lived in the Board and Care building — a living area for individuals who don't require as much assistance as those in other parts of our facility. Other than being confined to a wheelchair, Palmer bragged he was "as healthy as a horse." He valued his independence, and he said he'd rather die than be transferred to the Chronic Care Center where "the old and sick ones are." Palmer never did move because, while still a resident in Board and Care, he died in his sleep two weeks after celebrating his ninety-first birthday.

Residents and staff (especially staff) remembered Palmer as one of those persons who felt he should have a say in every aspect of how the nursing home was run: he instructed the dietary staff how certain meats should be prepared, and he made sure they knew which vegetables were better boiled or steamed; he informed those in housekeeping about the proper way to make a bed, telling them to be sure the corners were neatly tucked in; administration was told which of their policies concerning residents were out of date while, at the same time, advising them of ones that should be implemented; the nurses were informed they needed more training in regard to appropriate times when pills should be given out; nursing aides were given a lecture on how to give baths; the business office was advised that it needed to simplify the billing procedures and to print the billing statements in large print; the chaplain was advised as to the length of Sunday services as well as the necessity for brevity of prayers during noon-day meals. The need for short prayers, as Palmer explained, was because "long prayers make for cold food."

Palmer's primary focus, however, was on how the nursing home could save money. "After all," he would say, "it's my money. I'm paying for this place." In particular, his energy was spent in a personal crusade directed toward the overuse of electricity — he felt there were far too many lights left on unnecessarily. Every week Palmer wrote sharply worded notes to the administrator about "this terrible waste of *my* money." He even offered to submit a plan on monitoring the use of lights. "Saving electricity saves money," he pointed out. "Something has to be done," he had fumed. Palmer didn't mince his words in telling staff to turn off lights that (he thought) didn't need to be on. To carry out his campaign, he would wheel throughout the facility, turning off lights wherever he deemed it was necessary. It was rumored, though never verified, that lights were once turned off while a staff member was in a bathroom stall, leaving her in a "peculiar dilemma." Whether the story is true does not matter, for it became part of the Palmer legend.

One day, Palmer saw me coming out of my office. "Chaplain, ain't you going to turn off your lights?" he asked as he wheeled up and peered around me into my office.

"What do you mean?" I answered, pretending that I didn't know what he was getting at. I had hoped that by playing ignorant, he'd go easy on me.

"You're leaving your office, aren't you?"

"Yeah, I am." I realized that my ploy wasn't going to work. I thought about quipping that electricity is only penny cheap, but decided against it. Although Palmer had a sense of humor, when it came to his campaign, it was a different story. That he should "lighten up" a little was another quip that thankfully I decided it would be not wise to use.

"Ain't nobody going to work in your office while you're gone, are they?"

"No," I replied as I awaited my chastisement.

"Well, then," Palmer strongly suggested, "you should turn off the lights. You know, this whole place wastes too damn much electricity." He waved his arms around. "All these lights on around here. What do we need them on for?" His voice began to crescendo. "I wonder what the electric bill for this place runs for a year? Pretty damn high, I bet. Do you know how much the bill runs a year?" he screeched.

"No, I'm afraid I don't." I was trying to be very purposeful about keeping my voice calm while just wishing I could go back into my office, shut the door, and turn off the lights.

"I think I'll see the administrator about that; he should know," Palmer snarled and then warned. "He damn well better know since he's supposed to be in charge."

Without saying good-bye, Palmer turned his wheelchair and sped off in the direction of the administrator's office. As he wheeled away, I could hear him grousing, "Humph. Too many &*/#@*& lights on around here. &*/#@*& wasteful! Wonder what we pay a year? &*/#@*& administrator damn well better know …"

Right up to the day before he died, Palmer continued to search the facility for lights that, in his opinion, shouldn't have been on and were just "running up *my* electric bill." Staff would mention feeling Palmer's presence as they walked through a part of the building or entered a room and discovered switched-off lights that normally should have been on. Several months after Palmer died, the administrator and I were walking down a hallway leading to the Chronic Care Center. It was midmorning and, although light was coming into the hallway through windows, the overhead lights weren't on. We both knew that the ceiling lights needed to be on to provide the added illumination necessary for residents who are visually impaired. As the administrator flipped the light switch on, he glanced around, then looked at me, smiled, and winked. I knew what he meant and of whom he was thinking.

Just as the ghost of Palmer roams our facility switching off lights, Dottie's ghost makes the rounds seeing to it that staff are providing care to the residents in the manner of which she would approve.

Dottie worked at the nursing home as a head nurse for over thirty years before retiring. She later came back to live as a resi-dent when she was in her eighties. According to staff that took care of Dottie until she died, "the nurse in her" simply couldn't bear being away from the place. Those who knew her would tell you that she worried that no one could take care of the residents' needs in the way she knew they should be cared for, especially when it came to their bowel movements, or as she preferred to say, "their business."

From my conversations with those who worked with Dottie, she had earned the reputation as a head nurse for demanding nothing but perfection from her staff when it came to providing quality care for the residents. She would, for example, stand behind her staff and look over their shoulders to watch as a wound was dressed to make sure it was done properly. If it weren't done exactly the way she felt it should be, it would have to be done over. She would also give explicit instructions as to the correct way of taking a blood pressure or treating cuts and bruises. Since there were a number of residents who had difficulty swallowing because of strokes, she would have her staff crush all pills that were considered by her to be too large and therefore, might be difficult for older people to swallow.

One of her standard lectures was that crushed pills should be given with enough water, but better still, with a spoonful of applesauce. Dottie preferred the applesauce because, as she would tell her staff, it helped the residents do their business. According to her, if the residents did their business every day, they would be healthier and thus easier to care for while they were at the home. So staunchly did she believe that being healthy and doing one's business were inseparable that Dottie became obsessive about it when she came to live at the Home.

Those on staff when Dottie was a resident vividly remembered her obsessiveness. One nurse said, "Dottie was never quite sure if her own 'business' was adequate and often called upon me to check to see if it was."

A head nurse told me, "Dottie would peek around the corner of the door into the hall trying to get a nurse's attention, implying a request to come and look at her business. Once I assured her that it was adequate, she was pleased. A half hour later, however, she would be standing at her doorway again. This time she would have me check on her roommate's business to make sure it was adequate."

"And if it was?" I asked.

"Dottie would be assured then that her roommate was healthy and therefore, would have a good day. It was the nurse in her still taking care of residents. And you know, I continue to follow her policy today and I tell new staff to do it as well."

As a chaplain at the nursing home, I, of course, see staff give pills. I can't help noticing that the pills are crushed and are always given with water, or juice, and often, with applesauce. One day, while I watched a new staff person give a resident a crushed pill with a sip of water, a nursing aide instructed, "Be sure you have enough water. Even better, use applesauce. The residents prefer taking their pills with it. It's easier for them. Anyway, that's how I was trained when I began work here." When I heard the mention of applesauce, I thought to myself, Dottie would be pleased.

Those who consider themselves "the old timers" soon tell new staff about the ghost of Dottie. Along with the formal orientation staff receive about fire procedures, disposal of hazardous waste, staff benefits, scheduling, and all the other topics new employees expect to be told of, there is the informal orientation done by the old timers who knew Dottie. Besides relating the tale of Dottie and why she now roams the hallways, there is the opportunity for indoctrination whenever there is an unexplained event: Who picked up the soiled washcloth in Mary's room? Nobody knows. *Why, it must have been Dottie.* That coffee spill on the table in the nourishment room — who cleaned it up? *Dottie, of course.* And if there is some sound at night that you can't quite identify. *Well, it could only have been Dottie.* If you asked, where does Dottie live, the old timers would tell you that she lives "between the second and third floor of the Chronic Care Center." Why there? "Because that's the building where she lived as a resident before she died." But how can she live "between" the floors? "Because she's one of our ghosts."

Once a new staff person has been told the story of Dottie, administered crushed pills with a spoonful of applesauce and, most importantly of all, checked on the business of at least one resident to see if it was adequate, then the old timers are satisfied they can some day retire knowing that the legend of the ghost of Dottie will be passed on to the next generation of staff.

Palmer and Dottie's ghosts are friendly spirits, but more than that, they are caring spirits. And I, for one, hope they'll continue to make their presence known at our facility.

By the way, can you imagine what the conversation might be whenever Palmer and Dottie's paths cross?

"Dottie! Turn off those &*/#@*& lights! We don't need them on!"

"Now, Palmer, hush! How else are we going to see if Mary's business is adequate?"

The Gray-Haired Raggedy Anne

Imagine if you will, your wrist and forearm in a vise, and the vise tightened. Not to the point where it becomes painful, but where you know that you cannot extricate yourself without the vise's cooperation. The only discomfort you might feel would be some numbness in your hand and fingers. And, thankfully, once released, the only telltale marks are the vice's jaw prints that will disappear in time. As far as any lingering numbness, you only need to vigorously shake your hand to get the circulation going again. If you can imagine all of this, then you are ready for the next step: to move beyond the realm of imagination to reality. And the name of reality is Cora Belle.

Cora Belle has been a resident in the Chronic Care Center for eleven years. She is nearly 100 years old and weighs less than 100 pounds. Anyone walking past her, as she sits slumped in her wheelchair, could easily get the impression that here is a woman who is barely hanging on to life, an individual who is so weak that she would scarcely have the strength to hold a cup of coffee. This perception of Cora Belle seems to be confirmed as you gaze at her frail body. Eyes closed, and chin resting on her chest bone, she looks like a gray-haired Raggedy Anne doll whose stuffing is nearly gone. The only way you know there is life still left is that you can hear her mumbling to herself. You wonder, though, if she's even aware of her surroundings. As you walk by, however, *Raggedy Anne* suddenly comes to life and yells, "Com'ere." If, out of compassion, you respond to what you consider to be no more than a plea for help from a poor, weary, old soul, you're in for the surprise of your life. For as soon as you're within reach, your wrist and forearm are seized and locked in a grip that could only be compared to being in a vise.

My initial experience with Cora Belle coincided with my first week on the job as the chaplain. I was walking down the hallway of the first floor in the Chronic Care Center when I heard a yell, "Com'ere." I had noticed the woman when I walked by, but her head had been down, her face in her hands. It appeared that she was sleeping or, if not, off in her own little world and, I had assumed, didn't want to be disturbed.

"Hello, there. I'm the chaplain." No sooner had I introduced myself than her claw-like hands took hold of my arm and wrist. I was startled by her quickness and amazed at the strength of her powerful grip.

"What day is it, anyway?" she asked, her grip tightening. "You'd think that they would treat an old lady like me better. No one cares around here. They treat me like hell. Where can I get a cup of coffee in this damn place?" The words gushed out like water from a broken fire hydrant. "I don't remember how old I am, but I'm in my nineties. They don't have to treat me like they do. Can't get a decent cup of coffee around here. Food is cold. Why can't they serve some decent food around here? I've lost too much weight already. What day is it, anyway? I …"

"It's Thursday," I said quickly, knowing that I'd interrupted her, but needing to get a word in edgewise. "I'm sorry about your problems. I'll see what I can do," I offered, thinking that she would release me. "Why don't you let me go and I'll check about the food."

"Where am I anyway? How long have I been here? The food is terrible …" She was beginning her litany again without responding to my request. Her grip was as strong as ever as she continued. "Poor old lady like me shouldn't be treated like this. I don't have to live here. Is it raining out? When I came here, it was such a nice place. They served hot coffee. Damn fools; they don't know how to treat us old people. They think they can get away with anything around here. Do you know how old I am?"

"No, I don't," I interjected as I calculated how I could get her to release me. I thought about prying her hands off, but decided against that because I wasn't sure how she might react. Besides, I thought about how that might look to others — having the new chaplain in a wrestling match with a little old lady in a wheelchair, especially if she were screaming her head off. Admittedly, the thought also went through my mind that I might not have been able to pry her fingers loose. I shuddered at the thought of the staff witnessing a wrestling match where it was the chaplain who was screaming his head off. As she continued her rambling, I looked around for staff, but none were in sight. I was beginning to feel trapped. In addition, and it could have been my imagination, my hand felt as if it was getting numb.

"What year is it?" she asked, her grip as tight as ever. After telling her the year, she replied, "I was born in 1898, and I have always been two years older than the current year." After she mentally calculated her age, she exclaimed, "My gosh, I'm getting to be an old woman! I never thought I'd live this long; nobody in my family did. Damn fools around here. They don't know how to treat us old people. Can't even serve a hot cup of coffee ..."

It was only when an aide came to give her a cup of coffee and a cookie that she released her grip, and I slipped away. At the nurses' station, I asked one of the aides, "Who is that woman down there in the wheelchair?"

"Oh," she replied, chuckling, "that's Cora Belle. Did you meet her?"

"I sure did."

She grinned and then asked, "How's your arm?"

The next day I was wondering how I might help Cora Belle since she'd expressed a number of concerns. I decided to pay her another visit. She was sitting in the hallway just outside her room. As soon as I came within five feet she raised her head. "Com'ere," she yelled. I hesitated, but knowing she was hard of hearing, I moved closer and said hello. Her grip hadn't diminished in strength over the past twenty-four hours.

"Am I crazy?" she asked. "They think I'm crazy. Damn fools. I can't see without my glasses. They took them. How do they expect an old lady like me to see? What's for lunch? Staff don't care about me. I hope it's something I can chew. I've had a hell of a day. It's cold in here. How do they expect us old people to live here …"

Cora Belle went on and on and on, giving me little opportunity to respond. Having concluded that I could be of no help to her, I was just about to call for an aide and ask if she could be brought a cup of coffee, when Cora Belle suddenly released her grip, and said, "Thanks for listening."

The Enduring Human Spirit

What comes to mind when you hear the word Alzheimer's? The thought of a dreaded disease? A living nightmare? A silent prayer that it would never happen to you or your loved ones? Something you don't even want to think about?

What comes to mind when Alzheimer's is clothed with human flesh and you are reminded of a person (any person) who has this tragic illness? Someone who no longer has his or her mind? A person who deserves pity? One who would be better off dead? Someone who needs to be *locked up* for his or her own safety?

Finally, what comes to mind when Alzheimer's becomes personal and is used to describe a friend or a family member? A spouse who has become a stranger? A parent who has fallen into a black hole from which there is no return? A friendship that is lost forever?

Perhaps this disease has invaded your inner circle of family and friends. Words have failed you and you have only feelings — raw feelings where words no longer are adequate. As one wife, whose husband has had Alzheimer's for nearly two years, agonized, "There are no words to describe it; you only feel it. Every waking moment of every day you feel it."

Anger, embarrassment, guilt, fear, despair, grief, and profound sadness are some of the feelings that come when a loved one has

Alzheimer's. The feelings can be directed at many different people. Anger, for example, could be directed at the person with Alzheimer's, or at God, or even oneself.

The anguish this disease causes is reflected in the words of a woman I had coffee with one day. She talked about her husband who had died the week before. He had been a resident in the Alzheimer's Care Center at our nursing home. Though she visited him several times a week, he never acknowledged that he knew her. She told me that although it was difficult to have him die, she was not being overwhelmed by grief. The reason, as she explained, was because she felt as if she had lost him four years ago when he was diagnosed with Alzheimer's. His death was not easy for her, but as she shared, "It was only the death of his physical body. The person I knew to be my husband died a long time ago."

Connections based on past relationships such as husband and wife, parent and child, or sibling to sibling, often are no longer possible when Alzheimer's strikes. That is why it's so emotionally devastating to families.

Without minimizing the anguish experienced when a loved one has Alzheimer's, I would like to share some thoughts that invite you to look for the enduring, positive traits of the human spirit that still can be exhibited by those with this disease. I am aware that what I describe may not be applicable for all individuals who are afflicted with Alzheimer's. I also recognize the devastation one experiences when a loved one is lost to this illness.

The following vignettes from the lives of people with Alzheimer's reflect the genuine, indelible characteristics of what it means to be human. These personal examples are meant to help us recognize that, although this tragedy can rob persons of who they have been, as well as erase existing relationships, there are still meaningful attributes of the human spirit that survive to the very end. By looking for and relating to these traits, we still can be connected based upon the common humanity we share; often times, it's the only thing left. These points of connection exist in at least four different areas: humor, spirituality, the capacity to care, and the expression of appreciation or gratitude.

Most Alzheimer's residents still retain a sense of humor. While those with this disease may not remember people they had known all their lives, and though they may need step-by-step instructions on how to do the everyday things of life such as tying their shoes, or brushing their teeth, or unbuttoning their coats, there are some things they do not forget — and one is how to smile and laugh.

Ethel is a good example of a person with Alzheimer's who still can display a sense of humor. One day Ethel wanted me to meet a woman who was with her. It was her daughter, but Ethel simply referred to her as "the woman." Ethel introduced me as that "minister who comes to see me all the time." I talked to the two of them for a few minutes and then excused myself to go to a meeting. As I was walking away, I heard Ethel say to the woman, "He's such a nice man." I smiled to myself, but before I took another step, she added, "You wouldn't think he was a man of the cloth." I stopped and turned, and there was Ethel, grinning. I realized I had been expertly duped by a ninety-two-year woman whose illness may have taken away so much from her, but had not been able to take away her sense of play. Knowing Ethel, she'll hang on to her humor as tenaciously as she can as her way of saying, *I may not be the person I once was, but I still can remember how to enjoy the moment.*

Further evidence of the endurance of the human spirit within Alzheimer's patients is their spirituality. In each of the wings of the Alzheimer's Care Center, we have a weekly worship experience. Music plays an essential part, and the singing of familiar hymns such as "In the Garden" or "Amazing Grace" is important. Some of the residents can sing the words to an entire song while others only remember fragments. Others will hum, and one or two may even whistle the melody. When the Twenty-Third Psalm is read, some of the residents recite the words along with me while others will fill in key words, for example, when I say, "The Lord is my _____" and pause to let them finish the line. There was one individual who raced ahead of me, reciting the entire psalm by herself, and upon finishing, grinned triumphantly.

Even in times of crisis, when those with Alzheimer's feel that

God has abandoned them, there is the spirituality. Consider the case of Albina. "I've lost God," she said as she sat in a chair waiting for the worship service to begin. Her statement did not reflect any note of depression or despair. It was said matter-of-factly, as if losing God was just one amongst a number of things that she had lost along the way in life: a set of keys, a five-dollar bill, the grocery list, God. Yes, it is true that she is struggling with her spirituality, but the very fact that she is struggling shows her spirituality. It is quite common for people with Alzheimer's to no longer remember family and friends. While I have witnessed situations where the resident may not know someone as close as a daughter or spouse, I have yet to experience a person with this disease asking, *Who is God?*

The ability to express caring for others is seen in many of the residents with Alzheimer's and is another enduring trait of the human spirit. Merlyn, for example, has been a resident in the North Wing of the Alzheimer's Care Center for two years. He cannot verbalize his thoughts and he paces continually, no longer recognizing any member of his family; his behavior is often inappropriate. Many people might see him only as a poor lost soul who has lost touch with reality. If you spend any time with him, however, you'll see his expression of care for others — whether it be patting the hand of another resident who's crying, or picking up a magazine for someone in a wheelchair who dropped it. A staff person shared with me about a woman resident who held hands with a man who was crying as she walked up and down the hallway with him. Whenever staff approached the man, she shooed them away. Both of them are Alzheimer's residents. It was her way of saying, *Leave him alone. I know he's hurting. I'll take care of him.* This woman may not have understood where she was or what year or day it was, but she understood the pain of another and in her own way, tried to give comfort. I dare say that as she was reaching out to help another, she also was being helped by finding meaning and purpose.

The next enduring quality that those with Alzheimer's still are capable of demonstrating is that of expressing appreciation. Those with this disease who are able to communicate will often say thank you whenever something is done for them. They show a great appreciation of any kind of music. They'll appreciate the sun being out, or the coffee and cookies being served them, or a program presented for them by children from a nearby school. Their gratitude will express itself in so many different ways: a verbal thank you, a smile, or a nod of the head. John, a resident who is confined to a wheelchair, has expressed his appreciation by kissing the back of my hand and saying, "Thank you, thank you, thank you."

Why do people get Alzheimer's? Or, as I'm often asked, why does God allow such a terrible disease to be part of creation? Both of these questions are ones that I'm not able to answer. I can, however, extend an invitation on behalf of Ethel, Merlyn, Albina, John, and all the others like them: share and affirm within us those enduring qualities that still can bring us together in a common bond as human beings.

Questions for Reflection

These questions are meant to be catalysts, to stimulate creative thinking about ways at providing quality, holistic care for the elderly. In some instances, the reflecting may lead to new (perhaps untraditional) ways of providing care. Not all questions may apply to your situation, but *all* situations will benefit from reflecting upon them. Whether your community is a long-term care facility, a new retirement home, or the old neighborhood, you can adapt them to fit your situation.

The Wizard of Oz

1. Regulations and policies are necessary but they may sometimes get in the way of providing the best care for the elderly. For the purposes of discussing questions 1a through 1g below, regulations are defined as those "rules" that are external (state or federal laws). Policies are defined as internal "rules," that is, cre-

ated and adopted by the current living situation. Using the adjective *unfair* to refer to regulations and policies means that, in your opinion, such "rules" need to be reexamined because they do not serve the needs of the elderly.

    a. Make a list (no more than five) of regulations/policies that the elderly and/or their family members think are unfair.

    b. Make a list (no more than five) of regulations/policies that caretakers feel are unfair.

    c. Compare the lists in 1a and 1b. State your reasons why a particular regulation or policy is unfair.

    d. Of those listed in a and b, which ones are external?

    e. If you think a particular state or federal regulation is unfair to the elderly, what actions can you (or your facility or nursing home association) take to have it amended or changed?

    f. What current policies do you feel need to be reexamined because they get in the way of providing good care for people?

    g. If you are part of a facility, does it have a committee that reviews the policies affecting residents? If not, what would be the make up of such a committee? Consider forming one.

2. Sometimes people, whether elderly or not, make decisions that might not be in their best interest. To what extent do the elderly have the right to make these decisions? You can consider Herman's decision to smoke and compare it to Herman's decision to stay out in the storm.

3. When we label (stereotype) people, we tend to relate to them on the basis of the labels we have given them. Discuss how the following labels can affect interactions with and care for the elderly who are tagged as:

    a. Complainers

    b. Uncooperative

    c. A "behavior problem"
    d. Grumpy
    e. "Set in their ways"
    f. Other labels/stereotypes?

4. Once you have discussed how care of residents could be affected by the labels in question 2, discuss ways in which such stereotypes can be removed. The primary issues are
    a. How can we change attitudes toward people who have been tagged as "problems"?
    b. To what extent do the elderly have the right to continue to act as they have always acted? Does getting old mean we have to change our basic personalities to please our caretakers? Does getting old mean we can no longer learn to be better people?

5. Herman said that he was there to "add some color and character" to the place. Do you know people like that? What function/role do you think they play?
    a. Does your community encourage, discourage, or tolerate such "characters"?
    b. Is such behavior healthy or unhealthy for your community? Explain.

6. How do questions 2, 3, 4, and 5 tie in with dignity issues for the elderly?

Ghosts and Spirits, But No Goblins

1. Who are the ghosts/spirits in your community? What are the stories about them?

2. What kind of wisdom, insight, or truths do you find in those stories from question 1? (Dottie's ghost, for example, is concerned about staff providing the best possible care.)

3. Palmer felt he had every right to offer suggestions to those whose salaries he pays. What ways are set in place for your elderly to offer suggestions? How are they handled? How does the feedback get back to the suggesters?
   a. Who advocates for the elderly?
   b. Do advocates for the elderly have power and authority to make necessary changes?
   c. If you are in a facility, are staff and family members encouraged to be advocates for residents? In what ways? Do you feel you are one? Explain.

4. How much of a say should the elderly have in their care? What happens when a person's wishes come into conflict with staff goals? Who evaluates on a routine basis how care is delivered?

5. What official voice (for example, resident councils or senior citizen's groups) do your elderly have in your community? How are their needs addressed? Do they feel their needs are listened to? (If you are not sure, ask them.)

The Gray-Haired Raggedy Anne

1. Do the elderly expect all their problems to be solved or do they just want someone to listen? Discuss.
   a. Why is it important for them to be listened to?
   b. How does your community balance the needs of residents to be listened to against the needs of staff to get their work done?

2. In a facility, staff not only needs to listen to residents, but also to each other if they are to effectively work as a team. How are staff trained in listening skills? If you are a staff person, are you listened to? How does the question of listening apply to family members of the elderly? How does it apply to the elderly themselves?

3. Question to ponder: Is it possible to be listening to an elderly person all day long and yet not be listening? Discuss. What would be some creative ways to listen to the elderly so they know they are being listened to?

The Enduring Human Spirit

1. In what ways do those with Alzheimer's exhibit humor? Give examples.
   a. Would it be helpful for you to be given training in the therapeutic use of humor? Discuss.
   b. In what ways *does* your environment encourage humor and laughter?
   c. In what ways *could* your environment encourage humor and laughter?

2. What is being done in your community to encourage spirituality with those who have Alzheimer's? If you are in a facility without a chaplain, under which department would it be most appropriate to do this? Why that department? In the larger community, how can the spiritual needs of the elderly with Alzheimer's be met?

3. Expressing care and helping others encourages self-worth and meaning.
   a. Do you see expressions of this among the elderly you know? Share examples.
   b. Are there ways in which you can give your residents opportunities to be helpful to other residents and to staff? Be creative in this approach.

The advice of the aged will not mislead you.

— *Welsh Proverb*

As Time Goes By

"The clocks in this place are never right," Charlie complained to Ray as I listened. I had stopped for a few moments to chat, but for the most part found myself thoroughly enjoying just listening to their banter. Ray took another bite of his chocolate chip cookie and then looked up at the clock on the wall. After glancing over at the grandfather clock in the corner of the lobby, he nodded in agreement with his friend's comment.

Charlie and Ray, both residents on the first floor in the Chronic Care Center, were in the main lobby of their building, sitting in their wheelchairs, having coffee and cookies. Every morning they would wheel out to the lobby area and watch people come in and out of the doors leading to the parking lot. They said that it was their morning entertainment. Minutes earlier, they had received their midmorning snack from one of the volunteers who had come around with her cart distributing treats. Charlie was quite proud that he had been able to get *two* cookies each for himself and his friend instead of the one that was normally given out; he had bragged to us that it paid to turn on the old charm.

"Charlie," Ray asked with a puzzled look, "don't you think that they're trying to confuse us older people with these clocks?"

Charlie didn't respond to his friend's comment, however; the reason was because his attention was directed elsewhere.

"What are you looking at, Charlie?" Ray asked.

"Do you see that woman who just came in with the red coat?" Charlie answered, still not looking at Ray. "The one carrying a box of candy?"

Ray looked in the direction his friend was looking. I could see that he was squinting, causing his nose to wrinkle. "I see the woman," he exclaimed, "but I don't know if it's candy she's got. You know, I can't see as well as you. The doctor says ..."

"Ray, you already told me a million times what your doctor said," Charlie replied with a hint of irritation. "That *is* a box of candy," he argued and then added, "I think that woman is a relative of Ida's." He glanced over at Ray who was still squinting to see if his friend was right about what the woman was carrying. "You know Ida, don't you?" Charlie asked.

Ray scratched his head. "I'm not sure if I do," he answered with a puzzled look on his face.

"Oh, yes, you do," Charlie replied. "She's up on second floor in the room across from the nurses' station." When his friend still didn't seem to know, Charlie continued. "She's the one that comes down and sits over there by the bookcase. I think she's got glasses and always has on that same pink sweater."

"Oh, yeah, I know who you mean now," Ray answered. "And you think that's her relative?" he asked as he pointed to the woman carrying what his friend said was a box of candy. "So, what are you thinking about?" he asked Charlie.

I sat quietly, smiling to myself, suspecting what Charlie might be up to. *His sweet tooth was hungry.*

"Well." Charlie stretched the word out as long as he could without breaking it. "I might pay Ida a visit later on today. Maybe, after lunch." He grinned. "A piece of candy would taste good about that time." When he grinned again, his blue eyes twinkled. "Knowing her, she'll probably give me two."

"Get me a piece," Ray said. "Dark chocolate and one of those caramels." He glanced over at the woman. "Wait, maybe not caramel." He shook his head in disgust. "My dentures, you know," he explained sheepishly. "Better get me something with a cream filling, but make it dark chocolate."

"How will I know if it's cream?" Charlie asked.

"Just give it a little squeeze."

"I don't know about you two," I said, trying hard not to laugh. I thought of Charlie squeezing his way through the box of candy.

Ray turned to me. "Do you want Charlie to get you some, too, Chaplain? Charlie, get the chaplain a piece, will you?"

"No, no," I replied, "that's okay."

Both Charlie and Ray had the reputation of showing up wherever and whenever someone had food, especially sweets. Charlie was worse than Ray because he never would be satisfied with just one piece of candy or just one cookie. The staff had cautioned him about his weight, but he brushed them off, saying, "What else is there left for me to enjoy in life?" Besides, with the guileful ways Charlie used to satisfy his sweet tooth, he was also known as being quite the character and deservedly so. His reputation for the crafty ways he acquired things was only enhanced, for example, by how he obtained the fresh flowers he wore in the buttonhole of his sport coat every so often. It was no secret where Charlie got his flowers. Whenever a funeral spray was delivered to the front desk, Charlie was there, smelling the flowers and commenting on their beauty.

Ray looked at the clock again. "Charlie, don't you think they are trying to confuse us with these clocks around here?"

Charlie didn't answer because he was still watching the woman with the box of candy; she was now waiting at the elevator.

"Hey, Charlie!" Ray shouted. "Did you hear what I said?"

"What'd you say? What do you want?" Charlie replied as he watched the elevator's doors open and the woman in the red coat get on. Only after the doors closed did he turn toward his friend. "Now, what were you saying?"

"I asked if you thought they were trying to confuse us by having all the clocks around this place showing the wrong time." Ray paused to look over at the grandfather's clock in the corner. "No two clocks are the same. It's darn right confusing, don't you think?"

Charlie rubbed the side of his face, "Hell, what do you mean *trying* to confuse us? Those clocks never tell you the right time, but who cares. I don't even know what day it is anymore."

"It's Tuesday," replied Ray.

"Are you sure?" Charlie asked.

"Yup."

Charlie looked over at me and then back at his friend, Ray. "How can you be so sure?"

"Because they always serve chocolate chip cookies on Tuesdays," Ray answered with a smile. "All the other days they serve either sugar cookies or peanut butter cookies." He turned to face me. "Isn't that right, Chaplain?"

"I'm afraid I don't know, but I believe you if you say so."

Ray took another sip of his coffee. "I don't like the sugar ones because they fall apart when I try to dunk them."

"It's because you hold them in your coffee too long," Charlie chided. "I've told you that before. You never listen to me. You gotta dunk them; not drown them."

Charlie and Ray may not agree about cookie dunking but they both agree how confusing the clocks can be for them and the other residents. For reasons beyond my understanding, the clocks at our facility never seem to be right. Not only are they usually five minutes (more or less) off the correct time, but also, the numerous clocks in the various corridors throughout our buildings are seldom in sync. For example, the clock at one end of the corridor where Ray and Charlie live, may read nine twenty-seven while the clock at the other end of the corridor reads nine thirty-two.

"Hell, Ray," Charlie said, "don't matter what the clocks say around this place because we don't do much other than eat, sleep, and sit out here."

"I guess you're right," Ray answered.

Charlie and Ray's discussion about how befuddling it is to not know the right time brings to mind a stereotype that many people have of nursing home residents that does not do the residents justice. I have occasionally overheard visitors make the comment about how "these poor people" don't know what day, or month, or even year it is. (If they have seen the clocks at our facility, they probably know better than to include the time of day in their comments). The assumption behind their comments is that those who live in nursing homes, because of their age, have lost touch with everyday reality. While that may be true for the residents who are suffering from dementia, it does not apply to everyone. The fact is, for anyone who spends time within the same surroundings, having no pressing reason to live by the calendar or date book as the rest of the world does — the days, weeks, and months simply melt into each other, and one does lose track of time. This does not, however, apply only to the elderly living in nursing homes. I have, for example, taken young and middle-aged adults into a wilderness canoe area, instructing them to leave their watches at home. During the first day or two in the wilderness, many of these adults instinctively glance at their wrists, forgetting they are no longer wearing their watches. Toward the end of the second day and into the morning of the third, they begin trying to determine the time by the position of the sun. Before the end of the third day, however, and for the rest of the trip, most of them decide to stop living within the context of time and are content just to be. If you were to ask them what time of day it was, they would say it doesn't matter anymore. Furthermore, when asked about what day it is, they could tell you, but only after counting the sunrises they had experienced since the first day. Then there are those who, when asked about what day it is, simply reply they do not know nor do they care. These canoeists were people in their thirties and forties who had been without the *need* of knowing the time or the day for less than a week. Imagine how out of touch with "everyday reality" they would be after several weeks or months.

Not all those who live in nursing homes should be viewed as having lost touch with life just because they may not always know the time of day or even which day of the week or month it is. Charlie and Ray, for example, may not know nor care what time it is, but they can tell you when it is Tuesday — because chocolate chip cookies are always served on Tuesdays.

The next day I saw Ray sitting alone in the lobby. I walked over, said hello, and pulled up a chair. "Where's Charlie?" I asked, looking around for him.

"He's sick."

"Oh, no," I exclaimed. "What's wrong with him?" I was concerned because Charlie has had problems with high blood pressure in the past.

Ray laughed. "Don't worry, Chaplain. Charlie only has a stomachache. He ate too much chocolate yesterday."

The Hired Girl

The model of the 1909 wringer washer machine sitting on my office desk started Audrey reminiscing about the *good old days.* She had originally stopped in to inquire about the starting time for a particular program that afternoon in the chapel. Although she had planned to stay only long enough to get the answer to her question, the washing machine caught Audrey's attention, and I could see in her eyes the rekindling of long-forgotten memories. The washing machine, nicknamed by its makers, *The Hired Girl,* proved to be quite a catalyst as a conversation starter. Audrey was quick to point out how much better the wringer washers of yesterday were than the ones in our laundry rooms today. "It got the clothes a lot cleaner than what we have now because of the agitation action of the old machines." After Audrey finished making her point she went on to share other memories of growing up on the family's two hundred acre farm in the western part of Minnesota.

"Why, we had cows, pigs, chickens, and even a few horses," Audrey declared enthusiastically. "After feeding the chickens, I'd ride a horse to help herd the cows; that was such a good time." She looked at me with her head cocked, and a hint of a smile. "I bet you never pictured me riding a horse, did you?"

"Like a cowboy?" I asked, and then, correcting myself, "I mean, a cowgirl?"

"That's right, and I was only ten years old at the time," Audrey replied as she sat down in a chair and made herself comfortable. "I was too small to get up on the horse's back by myself so I would offer her a sugar cube. She sure loved those sugar cubes. That's why we called her Sweets." Audrey paused and closed her eyes for a moment as if she were picturing her horse and herself in bygone days. "When Sweets lowered her head, I'd climb on, and she'd just sort of toss me onto her back. I didn't have any saddle or anything, but we sure had fun. I chased those cows all over the place."

As Audrey talked about the hazards of riding bareback and herding cows, I tried to picture this white-haired, eighty-year-old great-grandmother who now hobbles around with the aid of a cane as a carefree young girl of ten riding her spirited horse called Sweets.

To encourage and invite people like Audrey to share stories of their youth is important because it serves a twofold purpose: 1) it gives them a chance to tell others about themselves, to feel that they have something worthwhile to share; and 2) it is truly rewarding to the hearer because, upon hearing the stories, one may begin to see, understand, and even relate to the person from a different perspective. For myself, I know I can no longer talk with Audrey without also remembering her riding bareback on her horse.

It's pleasing to those sharing the stories to know that they are being seen as individuals who have a history beyond the wheelchairs they are sitting in or the hearing aids they keep having to adjust. Certainly, there are some descriptions the elderly welcome; for example, being referred to as a grandparent or great-grandparent does give them a positive feeling about themselves and a worthwhile identity. On the other hand, they also may be pleased about being known as someone who could really dance up a storm when younger, or was a star athlete, or even, like Audrey, someone who herded cows while riding her beloved horse.

Looking at the model of the washing machine again, Audrey reminisced about the time she got her hand caught in the wringer and informed me that this was a possible hazard whenever one used a wringer washer. That it was a common occurrence was testified to by a number of visitors to my office who told about hands and arms getting caught in the "mangler" as some of them called it. One woman even told me that she got her hair caught in that "darn thing."

"We didn't have any fancy dryers in those days," Audrey said, as she continued with her reminiscing. "We'd hang the clothes out on the line. Nothing beats getting in bed underneath a sheet that had been dried outdoors." She closed her eyes for a moment and sighed. "Of course, I can remember looking out and seeing the laundry frozen on the line; we had to take it in frozen. You should have seen it. Pants and dresses were stiff as a board and we could stand them on edge. Mother stretched a line through the kitchen and let them thaw out from the heat of the potbellied stove." Audrey shook her head and smiled. "It didn't matter, though. The clothes still were fresher and cleaner-smelling than those coming out of the dryers we use now."

From that 1909 model wringer washer, Audrey went on to talk about homemade toys, her mother making dresses out of store-bought fabric, decorating a Christmas tree with stringed popcorn, being snowed-in on the farm, collecting eggs from the chickens, using an outhouse in the below-zero weather. Audrey admitted that she was remembering things she had not thought about for quite some time. It was enjoyable for both of us.

The other day there were three other visitors to my office and the model of the wringer washer caught their attention just as it had Audrey's. Since all three were in their mid-to-late twenties, however, only one could relate to it, remembering a grandmother talking about how she used one when she was younger. After sharing the story about Audrey and how it stirred some memories for her, I asked what should be sitting on my desk to stir their memories when they became eighty or ninety? Strange as it may seem, they couldn't think of one single item.

For Audrey it was a model of a wringer washing machine that opened up a floodgate of memories and stories. What do you think it will be for you when you're Audrey's age?

Appearances Can Be Deceiving

"Don't judge by appearances," Sophia yelled to the nursing aide who had just walked away after reprimanding her, but her words were to no avail. Perhaps if she had shouted louder, the aide would have heard and responded. However, at age ninety-three, Sophia's voice is as weak as the rest of her frail body. If she were able, it's quite possible she would have gone after the woman to confront her and demand an apology. Though Sophia felt she still had plenty of "spunk" left in her gas tank, she knew that spunk could not move the wheels of her wheelchair. She also realized she no longer had the strength of a few years ago when she could still wheel any place under "my own power." Now, unfortunately, her mobility is solely dependent upon others pushing her. "It's so hard to be dependent," she laments, "but what can I do?"

When I came upon Sophia a few minutes after her experience with the aide, she was staring down the corridor towards the nurses' station. The first thing I noticed were her eyes; they were filled with an intensity I hadn't seen before and appeared menacing as if a missile could be launched at any moment. Since Sophia is normally quite mellow and very pleasant to be around, I wondered what had raised her ire.

"What's wrong?" I asked. "You look a little upset this morning." I knelt down in front of Sophia and placed my hand upon her arm. Touching her was my way of signaling that I was a "friendly" and therefore, not the target for any missiles.

According to Sophia, an aide had come around the corner of the hallway just as Sophia coughed up something while clearing her throat. The aide assumed she had intentionally spit on the floor and had scolded her, saying, "Sophia, you shouldn't be spitting on the floor like that. A grown woman like you ought to know better." Sophia said that the woman, in reprimanding her, had used a tone of voice that normally might be used with a five-year old; not someone in their nineties. The aide walked away but not without warning, "Don't you be doing that again!" Sophia said that this woman hadn't even bothered to ask for any explanation. She had been so shocked by the aide's accusation that she was left momentarily speechless.

"I wasn't spitting," Sophia fumed. "I had something caught in my throat and I coughed it up. That was all that was to it, and she made it sound like ..." she paused to clear her throat. "I guess I still have some of it left." After unsuccessfully trying to cough up whatever she felt it was, she wiped her mouth with a tissue and looked angrily toward the nurses' station. "They just don't think about what they say."

"Do you know who it was?" I asked.

"I think it's one of those people down there," Sophia said as she raised her hand a few inches above the armrest of her wheelchair and pointed a bony finger. "I was clearing my throat. Just as I was doing it, this woman came around the corner and ..."

After Sophia finished retelling the story I looked at the three individuals standing at the nurses' station. One of the three had what looked like a resident's chart in her hands and was saying something to the other two. All three were smiling. Although I didn't say anything to Sophia, I wondered if they were talking about her. "Do you know which one of those it was?" I asked.

"How do I know which one?" Sophia replied. "Whoever it was, she stood in front of me so high and mighty. I couldn't look up to see her face because my neck muscles are so weak; it hurts me to look up. Humph! That woman thinks she can just hover over a person and say anything she wants. All she cared about was yelling at me for spitting. I wasn't spitting!" she nearly shouted. Sophia cleared her throat again before going on. "It was someone with white tennis shoes and wearing a white pair of slacks that had a black smudge on the right knee. I didn't see her face and I didn't recognize her voice." Sophia had to pause to take a deep breath. "I was too upset having someone accuse me of spitting." Her eyes narrowed. "I didn't spit! I was just clearing my throat. She came around the corner ..."

From Sophia's description, it was clear that one of the three women at the nurses' station could be eliminated. Even though all three wore white tennis shoes, only two of them had white slacks; the third was wearing a skirt.

The comment Sophia made about not being able to see the person's face made me realize how it must be for those sitting in wheelchairs and having people come up to them and speak to them without squatting or kneeling down. Her choice of the word "hover" to describe the person standing over her was an apt one.

Sophia's plea not to judge from appearances is one that certainly should be considered as a principle for all (staff, volunteers, visitors, and family) who have contact with those who live in long-term care facilities. It is also something that residents themselves need to be reminded of from time to time. The plea Sophia made is representative of others who are also concerned that they will not be judged unfairly. Here are some examples of other residents who would have good reason to echo Sophia's words:

Nora feels terribly embarrassed by the offensive odor that people might occasionally smell when they walk by her. Some, she says, will look upon her with pity while a few will view her with disgust as if to say, "Why can't she control herself?" She doesn't need pity or the other reaction. Instead, Nora wants people to be better informed about what it means when a person is incontinent.

Willis fell asleep shortly after the Bible study class began. After dozing for ten minutes, he woke up abruptly, looked around sheepishly, and apologized profusely, saying, "I'm sorry, I can't help it." The other residents in the room, however, didn't need an apology. They told Willis that they understood because it has also happened to them in other circumstances. Willis and his peers are not sure, though, that the younger generation always understands. The elderly are well aware of certain unflattering stereotypes people have of them. To provide a better understanding, Willis is quite willing to take the time to explain why he and others cannot help dozing at, what some may consider to be, inappropriate times.

Beverly, during meal times, often has more food on her bib and in her lap than on her plate. She is looked upon by some as a toddler in a high chair. If she could speak, though, she would tell you that she's had a stroke and has been working at feeding herself again. She could have someone feed her, and then she would appear clean and proper, but she is fighting to regain some independence. Beverly would like to tell you this, but the stroke has also affected her speech.

Vernon's glass of milk spilled onto the table and on his pants. He would ask you not to walk quickly past him, pretending as if he isn't there, because he would like to tell you about Parkinson's disease. During a visit, he held his hand in front of me and we both watched it shake until Vernon uttered words that no doubt would represent the feelings of many afflicted with this terrible disease.

"Look at that. I hate it when it does that. Damn thing is, I can't do anything about it. I hope people understand."

Nora, Willis, Beverly, and Vernon do not want to be judged by appearances. They are asking all of us to give them the chance to explain. Sophia would agree.

The Maxim

"Sometimes life is no more than putting one foot in front of the other," Henry had said to me one day as he acknowledged that he was losing the battle against failing health. He hadn't said it bitterly nor angrily, but rather, matter-of-factly. Knowing Henry, that didn't surprise me. It had been a maxim that he had lived all his life, and he knew the day he said it that it would be severely tested in the time ahead.

Henry had been a resident at the nursing home for nearly six years before he died. In all those years he lived at the Home, I never met another resident who had anything but respect and praise for him. For five of those six years, he was involved in every activity that was offered: he always had a front row seat whenever a movie was shown on the large-screen television set, he was the first to sign up for the annual cribbage tournament, and he always had two helpings of ice cream and cake at birthday parties. Whenever people gathered around the piano singing old-time favorites like *On a Bicycle Built for Two* or *I Want a Gal Just Like the Gal That Married Dear Old Dad,* Henry would be there, singing his heart out. It didn't matter to the others if Henry was off-key; they enjoyed his company, and his enthusiasm was contagious. If a group gathered in the coffee shop for a mid-afternoon snack and conversation, you could be sure Henry would be there offering to buy the cookies and to share a story or two. And if, upon the rare occasion, he didn't appear, the group would appoint someone to go and find him. If there had been a popularity contest, Henry would have won hands down because no other resident would have been foolish enough to try and run against him.

Henry's popularity was well attested since it extended beyond his peers. Whenever a local day care center made arrangements to bring a group of toddlers to meet the *grandpas* and *grandmas,* Henry always managed to have one or two of the youngsters sitting on his lap within minutes of their arrival. One of the memorable images others still have of him is seeing three-year-olds laughing and giggling as they gently bounced on his lap. As one of his friends observed, "That Henry; you can't tell who's having more fun." On more than one occasion, Henry was adopted as an honorary grandpa. And, if memory serves me right, one little girl cried sad little tears because she couldn't take him home with her.

In the first five years Henry lived at the Home, he experienced the usual aches and bouts of sickness but fortunately didn't face the more serious health problems that troubled many of the other residents. His decision to become a resident was brought about when a heart condition slowed him down and curtailed the amount of driving he could do. His doctor was concerned that the heart medication might affect his ability to drive safely. Since Henry had been volunteering at the Home for years, he decided that he should move into one of the areas where he could live as independently as his health allowed. I remember a conversation I had with him a week after he had moved in.

"I spent so much time volunteering here that I thought I might as well move in," Henry kidded as the two of us sat talking in the lobby of the Assisted Living area.

"Do you have any family?" I asked, trying to recall his family history.

"Well, Chaplain," he said and then sighed before continuing. "My wife died three years ago and Betty, my only daughter, lives in another state; her and I don't get to see each other much. My health is pretty good, but I figured that while I still had the choice, it'd be a good time to make the move. And I did."

I wondered if I would know when that time came for me, and if I did, I would have the wisdom and the courage to make the same decision. "Sounds reasonable to me," I said.

"Me, too," Henry smiled. "This way, I figure that I can still enjoy the place for awhile," he said, and then added with a chuckle, "before I get too old."

My eyes shifted to the cane that Henry had with him. "I like your cane," I said. His cane, which looked older than Henry, was beautifully carved with designs running from the grip to its end where the rubber piece for traction was attached.

"My father used it," Henry said, picking the cane up and showing it to me. "He got it from his father. My grandfather carved it. He said doing it gave him something to work on in his old age." When Henry chucked, it made me smile; he was always in a good mood and being with him made you feel happy. "I brought it with me the day I filled out the papers to become a resident here," he explained. "I thought it'd make me look like I belonged here." Henry smiled at his comment. "But, Chaplain, I want to tell you something. Can you keep a secret?" After I nodded, he glanced around to make sure nobody was within hearing range. There was only Art sitting about ten feet away from us, but we both knew that we could be shouting at one another and Art still wouldn't be able to hear us. Satisfied no one would hear, Henry confessed, "I really can get along without the cane. I just use it because I like the feel of it, but don't tell anyone. Okay?"

"I won't. It'll be our secret."

During that last year he was alive, though, the cane Henry used only because *he liked its feel*, became necessary for him just to keep his balance. After a stay in the hospital for what he jokingly referred to as "just one of my spells," his gait became even unsteadier. Other signs of the aging process became evident: he required more assistance for dressing and grooming himself; his occasional aches and pains became chronic; and worst of all, his memory began failing. For a man who prided himself in calling everybody by name, the memory lapses were very difficult for him. Within a relatively short time, it became apparent to everyone that Henry truly was failing. Up until then, his friends had hoped he was just going through some minor setbacks and that he would eventually bounce back and be himself again. That was not to be. His attendance at the group functions became sporadic. At times,

Henry simply would forget to come to the sing-alongs or for coffee. The main reason his attendance slackened, however, was as he told his friends, that he found it difficult to function socially. At first, he tried but found himself forgetting names of people he had known for nearly forty years. As much as those in the group tried to reassure him that they all have had the same experience, he knew (and so did they) that it wasn't just a momentary lapse of memory. Henry would begin to say something only, to his utter embarrassment, to lose his train of thought right in mid-sentence.

Although Henry never said, I suspect that another reason he had stopped attending the gatherings was to save his friends the awkwardness they might have felt in having to deal with his declining condition. A couple of months after the last time he had coffee with his friends, I stopped to talk to him. He was in the lobby sitting in front of the fireplace, staring into the flames.

"Hi," I said as I pulled up a chair.

"Oh ... ah ... ah ... hello there ... ah ... ah ... Chaplain."

"You've had it rather rough, haven't you," I said quietly.

"Uh, uh. Ah ... ah ... sort ... ah ... rough."

Henry knew exactly what I meant; I could see it in his eyes. We talked about the last few months and what he had been experiencing. He didn't express anger or self-pity, nor did he ever question why this was happening to him. He never implied that life was unfair. He had spent enough time at the nursing home as a volunteer to have witnessed others going through what he was now experiencing.

Shortly before his eighty-third birthday, Henry died. In that final year, his health drastically declined. Within a period of months he went from using his cane to needing a walker and finally, a wheelchair. During that whole time, however, he continued to try to live his maxim: "Sometimes life is no more than putting one foot in front of the other."

Questions for Reflection

These questions are meant to be catalysts, to stimulate creative thinking about ways at providing quality, holistic care for the elderly. In some instances, the reflecting may lead to new (perhaps untraditional) ways of providing care. Not all questions may apply to your situation, but *all* situations will benefit from reflecting upon them. Whether your community is a long-term care facility, a new retirement home, or the old neighborhood, you can adapt them to fit your situation.

As Time Goes By

1. Charlie and Ray talk about how confusing it is when the clocks in the facility are never right. That may be amusing on the surface, but it does not help their quality of life. With that in mind, discuss the following:
    a. In what ways do you think the places the elderly live make things more confusing for them?
    b. If you can't think of anything for 1a, ask some of your elderly acquaintances and their family members. When you ask, *just listen.* Don't make excuses, or become defensive. Make a list.
    c. Share the list from 1b with others concerned about the lives of the elderly. Don't dismiss the items listed as things that can't be helped or by saying, "That's the way things have always been." Think of creative ways to make things better.

2. The point is made in the story that people assume many of the elderly lose track of the day, month, and even the year, because they are confused. Environment can add to quality of life and alertness. Studies have shown that we are affected by our surroundings. If, for example, our surroundings are dull and lifeless, that will have a negative effect upon us.

    a. How can the place where an elderly person lives be improved to keep the person mentally alert? If you work in a particular part of a facility, how can you enhance your area both for the elderly you serve *and* yourself?

    b. What can be done to make facilities less "institutional"?

    c. Consider how the following may contribute to confusion in the elderly:

       1. Care providers using technical, medical terminology, or initials.

       2. No dress code for helpers or staff.

       3. Moving to a new place, whether it is from a person's home to a facility or between rooms in the same facility. (Who determines if the elderly person should move? Is it for the good of the person or because it is more convenient for the facility?)

       4. Changes in staffing.

3. Since meal times are important, one needs to evaluate the *total dining experience* as much as the food itself. An unpleasant dining experience not only takes away from an elderly person's quality of life, but it can also contribute to his or her confusion. With that in mind, consider the following questions:

    a. How much choice should the elderly have in selecting their meals? What are appropriate tradeoffs between nutritional requirements and preferred foods?

    b. Who should decide where the elderly eat? Who should decide who should be their companions at meals? If the elderly person is at a facility, how should the requirements of the facility be balanced with the needs of the elderly resident in choosing food, assigning seating, and selecting dining companions?

    c. Evaluate the ambiance of the dining experience. What is the noise level? What appropriate music might be played? Lighting? Decorations? How much "nursing" is done during meal times?

d. What would be the benefits of providing training for staff that prepare and serve the meals (training, for example, that is given to chefs and servers in the restaurant business)? How would that help make dining more enjoyable?

e. If you had to eat three meals a day where the elderly person you care about now eats, what would your expectations be in terms of service and ambiance?

f. In a facility, consider appointing a task force of staff, family members, volunteers, and residents to find innovative approaches for improving the dining experience.

The Hired Girl

1. Story telling is important to people. When we allow people to share stories, we learn something about who they are and what is important to them.

   a. In what ways do you encourage the elderly to share their stories?

   b. Discuss the statement: I don't have time to listen to their stories; I have work (or more important things) to do. How do you balance the tension between the two?

2. Medical charts are kept on all of us. They show only who the person is in terms of medications, wound care, etc. Discuss the benefits of having some pages in the chart about the persons themselves (photos of when they were younger, important events within their lives, etc.) How could family and friends be involved in this?

   a. If you think it would be worthwhile to have such pages, how could you go about trying it out on a limited basis as a test?

   b. How would you resolve the problem of confidentiality?

   c. Would keeping a memory book containing important events in the person's life be more effective because it

would be available for all visitors, not just staff?
d. What do you think the benefits of such pages would be?

Appearances Can Be Deceiving

1. How would you have handled Sophia's complaint about how the nursing aide talked to her?

2. What kind of policies do you follow to make sure the elderly have the ability to look nice? What could you do personally to help?

3. Nora is embarrassed when she has an "accident." How should staff, family, and friends help her?

4. In what ways do you take the initiative to educate others about people like Willis? What benefits do you see from having an outreach program to educate the community about aging? How would it help in a facility?

5. Beverly's dignity issue is at meal times. Should she be trying to feed herself? How should people helping her deal with the dignity issues involved in her eating?
   a. What are some things that helpers *should not* do while feeding a person?
   b. What would be some negative, non-verbal clues an elderly person can pick up from someone who is feeding them?

The Maxim

1. Henry enjoyed and was enjoyed by children. In what ways can you encourage intergenerational social gatherings? In what ways would a partnership between a facility and a nearby school or day care benefit both the elderly and the children? Who could investigate such a partnership?

2. Should the elderly volunteer? How can opportunities be made for continuing the volunteering experience even in facilities?
   a. List three *new* opportunities for the elderly to volunteer.
   b. Think of places where the experience of the elderly can provide important and useful information for the community as a whole.

3. How should the community help the elderly deal with aging-in-place issues? How should the community support the elderly when they need to move to places where increased care is available?

4. How do you deal with your own aging-in-place issues?

A friend is better than a thousand silver pieces.

— *Greek Proverb*

Old Friends

Recovering from surgery, Virgil was in a lot of pain. Two days earlier he had fallen and fractured a hip. Such an injury is an ever-present fear for the elderly because of its potential complications. The fall and resulting fracture was bad enough, but what made the day even worse for Virgil was missing the ceremony that evening. He was to be honored with a fifty-year service pin for his work in an organization he had belonged to most of his adult life. The staff told me that Virgil was so excited about the award that shortly after breakfast that day, he was already dressed in his best suit, asking their advice as to which tie to wear. Early that afternoon, and only hours before he was to be picked up by his escort, Virgil fell. He was later assured that the service pin would be sent to him. What could not be sent, I knew, was the memory of the experience he would have had of the ceremony itself.

As I walked into Virgil's hospital room, I was prepared to deal with a person who had every reason to feel down-in-the-dumps over his extremely untimely fall. Virgil, eyes closed, seemed to be resting comfortably. His shock of white hair, scattered in every direction, gave him almost a boyish look. As I walked over and stood by the side of his bed, I wondered what the consequences of this fall would be. A nurse once told me that so often in the elderly, a fall resulting in such a fracture could cause a person to physically decline quite rapidly. On the other hand, she had seen those who had bounced back from these things as if they were nothing more than a temporary inconvenience. She said that it is hard to predict how any person's healing will go. I wondered if these thoughts had crossed Virgil's mind. I was positive they had. He certainly had seen the worst outcome with many of his peers. Unquestionably, he was sharp enough to understand what he was up against. As I stood there, Virgil's eyes opened, and he smiled as he focused on me. I was just about to ask him how he was doing when he opened his mouth to speak.

"How ... ah ... is ... ah ... Stan ... doing?" He spoke in a whisper. His mouth, dry from the pain medication, made it difficult for him to form the words. "He ... ah ... wasn't ..." Virgil paused and motioned toward his water glass. After I held it for him so he could take a sip with the straw, he motioned for me to put it back, as he tried again to speak. "He ... wasn't ... ah ... feeling ... too ... ah ... good ... before ... I ... came ... in." Virgil asked for another sip of water before finishing. "Think ... he ... had the ... flu ... or ... something."

Virgil considered Stan a friend, and for Virgil, friendship was more important than receiving an award, or even being worried about his own medical problems. Stan felt the same about Virgil and, after learning I had been to the hospital to see his friend, made it a point to look me up the next day to ask about Virgil. Stan's flu turned out not to be flu at all, but rather a recently diagnosed inoperable tumor that was spreading. The doctor had told him that the tumor had spread too fast and that there wasn't much they could do. Stan, however, wasn't as concerned about the cancer as he was about his friend. He made sure I promised not to tell Virgil about the tumor. Stan wanted the news withheld from Virgil because he didn't want his friend to worry about it while in the hospital. He had planned to share the news over a cup of coffee with Virgil the day after he had been honored with the fifty-year service pin. Now, as far as Stan was concerned, it would have to wait until Virgil got better. He would tell him then. Maybe.

This bond between Virgil and Stan reminded me of the time when I, as a young child, went with my grandfather to see someone he had not seen in many years. Apparently, they had known each other as young men, but they had gone their own ways and had lost track of each other until my grandfather was told that this person was in town visiting some friends. Now their paths were about to cross again. My mother said that they both were from "the old country." At the time, all I knew about what the old country meant was that it was far away across the ocean.

Holding hands, my grandfather and I walked toward the door. Before we even got there, it opened and a balding, gray-haired man came out. The two looked at each other for a moment and then did something I still can picture: they embraced, kissed each other on the cheek, and uttered but one greeting to each other, "Friend."

Both Virgil and Stan have since died as has my grandfather, but their stories bring a richer, deeper meaning to the expression "old friends."

A Luncheon Date

"It's really weird," the nursing assistant said to me as soon as I walked up to the nursing station.

I was just beginning to make my rounds to visit residents on the third floor of the Chronic Care Center. The expression on this staff person's face told me that something was troubling him as he continued without waiting for me to respond. "Clarence is going to eat lunch in the room with his dead wife. Isn't that weird?"

One may agree with the nursing assistant's reaction to the husband's desire to have a meal in the same room where, an hour earlier, his wife had died and where now her body still lay. Before you make your judgment on Clarence's decision to have lunch with his wife, let me provide you with some background information that might help you see the situation from Clarence's perspective. After you hear me out, then you can make your own decision as to whether this whole scenario should be classified as being weird.

Clarence's wife, Mary, was at a point in her declining physical condition where she was receiving from the staff only what is called *comfort care*: her mouth would be kept moist using cotton swabs; her frail body positioned to help her breathe more comfortably; pain relievers would be given whenever needed. The doctor had declared that there was nothing more that could be done; her body was shutting down, and the best the staff could do now was to make her as comfortable as possible. Her shallow breathing, unresponsiveness, and falling body temperature all were indications that the end was near. Clarence was called during the night when the staff judged that his wife could die at any time. He had spent the rest of the night with her as he dozed off and on in the chair next to her bed. That morning, staff called to inform me of Mary's condition and that her husband, who was with her, would no doubt appreciate a visit. I stopped in and, after talking with Clarence about all the good memories he and his wife had shared, we had a prayer together. He had asked me if I could pray that she could go quietly and quickly so that she wouldn't have to suffer any more. It wasn't an easy request for him to make as he held her limp hand and stroked her hair.

"We've been married fifty-three years," he said after I finished praying. He looked at me and said it again but this time in a whisper, "Fifty-three years. It may seem like a long time but it goes pretty fast. It seems like only yesterday." I could only nod my head as I noticed the tears running down his cheeks.

After visiting for a few more minutes, he thanked me; and as I got up to leave, he returned to his chair to resume the vigil. I hadn't been in my office longer than fifteen minutes when the phone rang. It was a nurse calling to let me know that Mary had just died. When I arrived at her room, Clarence was sitting in the same chair holding her hand, tears freely running down his cheeks. As I came in, he stood up, and we hugged as he said quietly, "She's gone. She's at peace now." We talked about their years together and how special they were; how she was so much part of his life. He told me that the service would be in their hometown, and people from the funeral home would be coming down to take her back.

"How long will that be?" I asked.

He looked at his watch. "It's going to be about three hours before they arrive," he replied. When asked what he planned to do during that time, he said, "Oh, I'm going to stay with her until they get here."

"We had a prayer together and I left, closing the door behind me so that Clarence and his wife could be together. It was an hour later when I was up on the floor again to see another resident that the nursing assistant made the comment, "It's weird," and then informed me about Clarence's decision to have lunch in the room where the body of his dead wife lay.

Upon hearing where and in what circumstances Clarence was eating lunch, some might consider it weird. Others, perhaps, might even think of it as being spooky. I would hope, however, that the whole situation could be seen from another perspective. Clarence and his wife shared many things in their fifty-three years together and, for him, having this quiet time and a meal with the woman he loved so much would be very appropriate. One might even walk by the closed door during this time and hear him talking to her. For those of you who might think that would be weird, perhaps some time spent at a cemetery would change your mind. It's not uncommon to see someone standing by a headstone talking to a loved one. Nor is it uncommon for people to have "conversations" with a loved one who has died. You or someone you know may have had such a conversation as well.

Clarence and Mary had known each other for close to sixty years. During that time their friendship and love bonded them in such a way that one, usually without being told, often knew what the other was thinking and even how the other would respond to a given situation. They were together, as Clarence told me, "in good times and in some pretty rough times, but we made it together." Just as they shared life, Clarence, in his own way, was sharing with Mary, her death.

He stayed because he did not want her to be alone in those hours until the funeral director arrived. Having lunch with her was just another expression of his love and devotion.

Friends for Life

"Aghhh ... Let ... me ... aghhhh ... go," Alfred screamed as if his very life was being threatened. "You're ... not ... me ... back ... aghhhh!"

Even though Alfred was nearly slipping out of his wheelchair, he continued to hang on to the edge of the hallway door with a strength well belying his eighty-five years. With one hand clutching the door handle and the other having a firm grip on the edge of the door itself, he was prepared to make his stand. He was determined not to go back. Not now. Not after he had come this far.

Two nursing aides had been sent to bring Alfred back to the third floor of the Chronic Care Center where he was a resident. The aides had caught up with him in "the ramp," a first floor hallway that connects the Chronic Care Center to another part of the facility that houses the Assisted Living apartments, the Chapel, and what is known as Town Square.

Halfway down the ramp where Alfred was at the moment are two fire doors, doors that automatically close whenever the fire alarm sounds. It was one of these fire doors that he had latched onto, tenaciously refusing to let go. The aides tried to persuade him to return to his room but were not being very successful. Alfred was becoming more belligerent by the moment; the aides, more desperate.

"Alfred, you've got to come back, please," pleaded one of the aides, looking to his partner for help.

"Aghhh ... no ... nooo!" Alfred cried, looking at them as if they were the enemy; in his mind, they no doubt were.

Since neither of the aides had the time to spend escorting Alfred wherever he had decided and was determined to go, they didn't relish the unpleasant task that lay before them. They looked at one another and nodded their heads knowingly; both knew that it was a difficult situation as they talked quietly between themselves about what their next move should be.

I heard the yelling from my office and went to investigate. When I came upon the scene, Alfred was still hanging on to the door and the two aides were still trying to prevail upon him to return to his floor. As I was later told, one of the aides had initially attempted to turn Alfred's wheelchair around. This action prompted his yelling and grabbing hold of the door. The aide, startled by the outburst, quickly let go of his wheelchair. From that point on, if either of the aides got too close, Alfred wildly kicked out at them. He wouldn't listen to their explanation that they were responsible for him and they needed to bring him back.

Alfred, as he later told me his side of the story, had managed to get down to the first floor by sneaking onto the elevator. He had wheeled up to the elevator doors where he lived on the third floor and just waited. He didn't have to wait long before the doors opened, letting some visitors off. When the visitors got off, Alfred wheeled on. Once he was on, he figured he was home free.

As soon as Alfred got on the elevator, however, the staff were alerted immediately when an alarm sounded at the nurses' station. A device called a Wanderguard that Alfred wore on his wrist had activated the alarm; it is an electronic wristband that many residents wear. When Alfred got on the elevator, a circuit box located on the wall by the elevator doors picked up the signals from his electronic wristband. Once the signals are detected, it activates an alarm at the nurses' station that buzzes quite loudly. The wristband is for resident safety. Those residents, like Alfred, who are apt to wander without regard for their own well-being, wear it. The danger is that residents may not only leave the floors where their rooms are, but also, if given the opportunity, the facility itself.

Being in a wheelchair is not a deterrent to a resident who is determined to leave the building. One day, as I was leaving work, I came upon a resident in his wheelchair who was outside in a temperature of thirty degrees. This man wore slippers but had no socks on and was dressed in slacks and a short-sleeved shirt. Although shivering and complaining about being a little cold, he was still headed away from the building toward a busy main road. He was disoriented and sufficiently confused not to have been able to return to the building himself. He wasn't wearing an electronic wristband and, as we now know in hindsight, should have been. The very next day this man received a Wanderguard. I was reminded of him as I was dealing with Alfred now.

"What's going on, Alfred?" I asked in a light-hearted tone while signaling to the aides that I would stay with him and they could go.

Both aides were grateful and looked relieved as they said their good-byes to Alfred while informing me they needed to go back and attend to their other duties. Having thanked them for their concern about Alfred, I assured them that I'd see to it that he would be brought back to the third floor.

"See you up on third, Alfred," one of the aides said as he looked back and waved; the other aide simply smiled and waved. It was obvious that they cared about him even after having gone through such a trying experience.

"Not ... aghhh ... going ... good-bye," Alfred yelled. "I ... aghhh ... good-bye ... see ... you." He didn't wave but hung on to the door until the two of them were gone. It was only after the aides turned the corner of the hallway and were out of sight that Alfred loosened his grip.

"Shall we go for a little ride?" I asked. After he nodded yes, I began to slowly push his wheelchair in the direction he had been originally headed.

"They ... he ... go ... aghhh ... damn ... not ... nurse ... room ... I ..." Alfred's response still showed a great deal of agitation. The agitation, I suspected, was a combination of his being upset about what had just taken place as well as a high level of frustration on his part from not being able to verbally express himself the way he wanted. If he could have expressed himself, perhaps none of this would have happened.

Alfred had had a mild stroke two months earlier that affected his speech. His stroke, along with increasing signs of memory loss and resulting confusion, had precipitated his move to the Chronic Care Center. The move had been difficult for him because he had left friends behind in the Board and Care building where he had lived for over two years. He was determined to return to his previous living area, and had worked very hard with the speech therapists. Through weeks of therapy he learned to communicate. By concentrating and speaking slowly, Alfred could verbalize his thoughts; what came out might be a little choppy, but was reasonably understandable. Unfortunately, his sentences would become garbled and disjointed whenever he became agitated.

"Do you want to go down to the coffee shop and see who's there?" I asked. "Perhaps we could look around at some of the stuff being sold, and we might even run into someone you know.

Wouldn't that be nice?"

"Yes ... ah ... yes," Alfred replied, nodding his head in agreement. He was calmer now, knowing that he wasn't going to be taken back to his room.

When Alfred and I got to the area outside the coffee shop (an area called the Promenade), we discovered that it was being used to host the "birthday of the month" party for those residents who lived in Assisted Living and Board and Care. Tables had been set up, and cake and ice cream were being served. There were close to a hundred residents in attendance; they had come to celebrate the birthdays of a dozen or so of their peers.

Alfred's friends and former neighbors immediately recognized him. As I wheeled him around, going from table to table, many greeted him with a warm smile and a hearty handshake.

"Hi, there, Alfred," a petite, silver-haired, attractive woman called out in a friendly voice; it was Mabel, one of his good friends.

"Nice to see you, Alfred," another said.

"We miss you," Milton exclaimed as he wheeled his wheelchair up to Alfred. "When are you coming back? Soon I hope."

"Oh, look," Bob exclaimed to the group at his table, "there's Alfred." He, along with the others at the table, raised their cups of coffee in a toast.

Alvin hollered and waved at Alfred from across the way, offering him a welcoming smile. "You're looking great, my friend."

Besides the verbal greetings, there were handshakes, pats on the back, and even a few hugs. The effect upon Alfred was amazing as he smiled and laughed; all signs of agitation were gone.

Although his sentences were still a little garbled, his friends were able to understand him. Any confusion now was only because of his excitement at seeing his old friends.

After Alfred and I had spent time visiting with his friends, we went into the coffee shop to browse in the general store. After some time passed, I knew I needed to return to the work I had been doing before getting involved with Alfred.

"Alfred, are you ready to head back home?" I asked.

"Uh huh," he replied.

All the way back Alfred and I talked about how gratifying it was for him to see his friends. I told him that he had so many people who cared about him. To each of my comments, Alfred would smile and say, "Uh huh, yes." When I wheeled him past the spot where he had, just a short while ago, hung on so desperately to the door and fought with the two aides, I wondered if it would trigger something within him that would cause him to balk at going back to the third floor. We went past the two fire doors, however, without any indication from Alfred that that had been the spot where he had made his stand.

"It's been a great time," I said to Alfred as I pushed the button for the elevator that would take us back to the third floor. He nodded his head in agreement. We both knew that he had set out to see his friends, and he did it. He was content.

Alfred never returned to live in Board and Care but every so often, the alarm buzzes at the nurses' station on the third floor of the Chronic Care Center. When it does, I suspect it might be Alfred on his way to see his friends again.

Always Aim for the Bull's-eye

"Nobody understands the pain I feel being in this wheelchair," Harold had said to no one in particular even though I was in the room with him. We were looking out the window, watching a young man push a wheelchair — probably a grandson spending time with his grandmother. Both were experiencing the pleasures of the autumn colors as the wheelchair slowly moved along the walkway encircling the facility. A slight chill was in the air, lingering from the overnight frost, and the maples and oaks were releasing orange and gold-colored parachutes that floated gently to the ground. Every now and then, the young man would bring the wheelchair to a halt, retrieve a newly fallen parachute, and place it on his grandmother's woolen lap blanket for her to examine. Although Harold and I were not privileged to hear their animated conversation, it was obvious that the two were enjoying themselves on that sunny afternoon in late September.

With the changing of the seasons, Harold knew that the arthritic pain in his knees would change as well, going from moderate to severe, depending upon the harshness of the winter. He and many of the other residents who also suffer from arthritis would tell you that they could feel it in their bones whenever the weather changes. Harold was in constant pain from the unsuccessful knee surgery he had had several years ago. He had maintained that the operation served no purpose other than aggravating his arthritis. On that day as we gazed at the world outside his window, his comment, I sensed, was not intended to refer to physical pain.

In his mid-eighties when he died, Harold had been a resident for nearly five years; the last three of those years being confined to a wheelchair. Before his knee surgery, Harold had been a fairly active resident, using a walker to get around. One of the ways he kept himself busy was volunteering as a tour guide for visitors; he knew his way around the spacious buildings better than some of the staff. Since he was considered by everyone as *Mr. Public Relations*, he was especially sought after as a guide for those individuals who were considering the Home as a possible place to live. Those who were given the tours, having been totally charmed by Harold's humor and wit, often remarked at the tour's end that they were ready to move in tomorrow, provided, they added with a laugh, that their tour guide would still be there to show them around. Even after Harold was forced to trade his walker in for a wheelchair, he continued to give tours, though not as extensive.

Outgoing and quite articulate, Harold was considered an ideal spokesperson for, as he would say, "the old folks." Once, when a staff person mentioned to him that she was attending a conference on gerontology, his comment was, "Take me along. I'm an expert on it." On another occasion, I overheard one of the housekeepers ask Harold how old he was. "I'm old enough to remember everything," he replied, giving her a wink as he wheeled away.

Having had the reputation in his working days of being a hard-nosed business executive, Harold was someone who could intimidate both residents and staff alike. He would, though, exercise his forceful style on other residents only upon rare occasions, and only with those who he felt were being unreasonable in their demands. His pet peeve was with residents who were concerned only that their individual needs were met first and who didn't consider the needs of the residents as a whole. "The *me first* attitude," Harold would dryly observe, "doesn't only belong to the younger generation."

Harold may have gained a few detractors in his way of handling things, but he was genuinely admired and respected by all the other residents as a champion for their rights and general welfare. It was mainly for staff, especially those new on the job, that Harold reserved most of the intimidation he wielded. More than a few of them referred to him as the bulldog-in-a-wheelchair, a description Harold gladly fostered to strengthen his tough-guy persona. Although the new employees, upon their first encounter, didn't know how to react to him, they quickly learned that Harold's gruff exterior was simply his way of testing them to see if they "were worth their salt." If he judged they were not, he advocated that either they be asked to leave, or at the very least, receive additional on-the-job training. To be sure that some kind of action was being taken on his recommendations, Harold would routinely stop by the administrator's office to visit, and would continue his visits until the issue had been resolved to his satisfaction.

Harold said to me one time when we were talking about staffing, "These are the people who are responsible for taking care of my friends here, so they better know what the hell they're doing." He had shared this comment after he had complained to the charge nurse about a certain staff person who he felt was rather rough with another resident as she was transferred from her wheelchair to her bed. The resident, who happened to sit at the same table with Harold during an activity, had told him about her terrible experience.

Harold often spent time wheeling up and down the hallways

"practicing his quality control." He once upbraided a member of the staff he had personally witnessed being impatient with a resident. When the staff person complained to her supervisor about Harold's interfering with her duties, Harold was asked to give his side of the story. After listening to Harold for a few minutes, the supervisor thanked him and then called the employee back to be reprimanded. The resident in question was a stroke victim who could not speak for herself. "I just couldn't stand by and watch my friend being treated like that," Harold said. Interestingly enough, although Harold referred to the resident as a friend, he personally didn't know her.

Once new staff survived the initial encounter with Harold and his rough exterior, most of them came to understand him. If he was surly with them, his motivation was that he wanted to make sure the residents' needs were properly being attended to in a professional and caring manner. Staff may not always have appreciated his yelling, and they certainly were not pleased with Harold's reporting them to their supervisors for what they considered minor things, but they did recognize that he was a strong advocate for residents' rights. Even those who didn't agree with him respected this bulldog-in-a-wheelchair for his unyielding efforts to make sure residents received the utmost of quality care. Considering his tireless advocacy, many agreed that Harold was the best friend the other residents had at the home. As far as he was concerned, if it meant he had to act like a bulldog at times, so be it. That his bark was worse than his bite was something that he wanted to keep as secret as possible. Of course, that was the worst kept secret at the Home.

There was another side of Harold that offset the bulldog image, and that was his sense of humor and unyielding zest for life. The coming together of these two traits of his personality, in any given set of circumstances, produced some worrisome moments for staff. For example, soon after Harold received his wheelchair, he wheeled down the hallway of the first floor where he was a resident, until he reached what had become known throughout the facility as "the ramp." The ramp is the connecting hallway between the Chronic Care Center and the building that houses an area called Town Square.

The ramp is the only access if one wants to travel from the Chronic Care Center to these other parts of the facility; it had been the only possible design solution to provide the connecting link. Unfortunately, the design required an incline, sloping down from the Chronic Care Center into the Town Square area. The incline causes those in wheelchairs to pick up enough speed that, if left unchecked, can present a problem. To alleviate this, handrails were installed on both walls of the connecting link for residents to use. If residents choose not to use the handrails, they still can control the speed of their wheelchairs by dragging their feet or gripping the wheels as they use their hands to control the speed. Many residents in wheelchairs find the return trip back to the Chronic Care Center easier, even though it means going up the ramp. Though strenuous, they pull themselves up by use of the handrails, or turn their wheelchairs around, and go up backwards, using their feet to push.

My office is located in the Town Square area, almost directly opposite the bottom part of the ramp. If you were to come down the ramp and veer slightly to the left in your wheelchair, you would roll straight into my office. Since I always have my door open to make it easier for residents to have access, I have an unobstructed view of the entire ramp. Many times I have watched residents sit in their wheelchairs at the top of the ramp, apparently contemplating whether they felt venturing it was worth a cup of coffee at the coffee shop or a movie at the cinema. Most of them decide it is, and cautiously come down hanging on to the handrails on the wall. After they reach the bottom, often they breathe a sigh of relief, and a few of them even raise their fists in triumph or give me the thumbs-up sign for victory.

While other residents in wheelchairs may look upon the ramp as a necessary evil, Harold saw it not only as a challenge, but also as a great opportunity to test his zest for life. Harold would wheel down the hallway from his room until he came to the top of the ramp. He then paused at the top, looking down the forty-foot slope much like a ski jumper pauses before beginning the run. In his pausing at the top, Harold was not mustering his courage, but rather, with a grin on his face, merely glorying in the moment. Unlike other residents who slowly inch down the ramp, when Harold felt it was time to begin the descent, he would aim his wheelchair and push off. Without using his hands or feet to slow his wheelchair, Harold would pick up speed, grinning all the way, and letting forth an enthusiastic "Wheee!" Just as he got to the bottom, he would put his feet on the floor and come to an abrupt stop. He often bragged that he could stop on a dime if he had to.

As I sat at my desk one day, I looked up to see Harold at the top of the ramp. It was mid-morning, and I knew that he was making his daily trip to the coffee shop to have a donut and to visit with his friends. He shoved off as usual, but this time he came down the ramp so fast I was concerned he wouldn't be able to stop.

"Whoa, Trigger," Harold yelled after coming to a halt.

"Someday you are going to crash into my office," I yelled out to him as he came closer.

"No chance," he said with a laugh.

"Tell you what," I suggested. "Why don't I paint a bull's-eye on the wall next to my door. That way, you'll have something to aim for, and I won't have to worry."

"Let's do it," Harold said in a tone of voice that made me question whether he realized I was joking. He said he did, but I know he would still have considered doing it, if only to add a little spice and fun to the lives of the old folks. Knowing Harold, if it had been possible, he would have had that bull's-eye painted on the wall and made it into one of the tour stops.

Much to the consternation of staff, Harold's sailing down the ramp inspired other residents in wheelchairs to try it as well. Eventually, Harold was giving encouragement to those who had never gone down alone, to conquer the ramp rather than have it conquer them.

A year after Harold and I had watched the grandson place some autumn leaves upon his grandmother's lap for her to look at and touch, Harold died quietly in his sleep. He is still missed by residents and staff, but one of the legacies he left behind to all his friends at the nursing home was to be sure to always aim for the "bull's-eye." They understood that, for Harold, the bull's-eye was a metaphor for living life to its fullest, even when it meant you had to do it in a wheelchair.

Since Harold never explained it, I have often wondered what prompted the comment he made that September day when he said that nobody understood the pain he felt being in a wheelchair. Was it his way of acknowledging that he knew he would never again be able to walk among the autumn leaves? Perhaps it was the sober realization that while he had the attitude and playfulness of a person sixty years younger, his physical body was rapidly failing him. Or was he worrying about who would be an advocate for his friends after he was gone?

The bull's-eye was never painted on the wall, but those who knew Harold can see it whenever they come to the top of the ramp and look down.

Questions for Reflection

These questions are meant to be catalysts, to stimulate creative thinking about ways at providing quality, holistic care for the elderly. In some instances, the reflecting may lead to new (perhaps untraditional) ways of providing care. Not all questions may apply to your situation, but *all* situations will benefit from reflecting upon them. Whether your community is a long-term care facility, a new retirement home, or the old neighborhood, you can adapt them to fit your situation.

Old Friends

1. Virgil was about to experience a significant event (receiving an award). There are significant events within the life of each of us (birthdays, anniversaries, births of grandchild and great-grandchildren, receiving awards and recognition, anniversary

of when we entered a facility, etc.).

    a. How do we celebrate (besides birthday parties) the lives of the elderly? How could we celebrate them? Discuss celebrating the life of a person each week until all people in your community are celebrated.

    b. How could recognition (la) enhance the quality of life for the elderly?

    c. Discuss having such recognitions as part of a resident care plan in a facility.

2. Define and then discuss what is meant by holistic health care. What would that mean for the elderly and their caretakers? Take a survey of the elderly, their families and their caretakers to determine:

    a. If they think the present system of care is based on a medical or a holistic model.

    b. What model would they prefer to work under?

    c. What things could be done to develop the system of care you prefer?

    d. How do the groups view the situation the same way and how do they view it differently?

3. A holistic model of health care means, in part, that health care providers work as teams and that providers from all areas are partners. With that in mind, discuss the following:

    a. How well does teaming work in your care team? What could be done to improve it? How could *you* improve it?

    b. Teamwork means good communications. In what ways could communication be improved among providers? What could *you* do to improve communications?

    c. How can communication between providers and the elderly be improved?

4. How does your community encourage friendships among the elderly? What programs are in place that bring the elderly

together in intentional ways (hobby clubs, etc.)? How can friendships be maintained when the people are separated because of illness or disability?

5. In a facility, how should staff be involved in helping residents visit with friends in other parts of your facility or outside of the facility? How could they help two residents stay in touch if both were bed ridden?

6. In what intentional ways do you promote a sense of belonging among the people who reside in your community? Do health care providers feel they are part of that community? If there is not a sense of belonging, how could you promote it within the community as a whole? Within your own area?

A Luncheon Date

1. What kind of training should be given to health care providers in dealing with death issues? Inquire as to what kind of training they would like. Who could give that training?
   a. In a facility, are the policies concerning death geared toward facility needs or family needs? For example, the facility's need to have a room cleaned out for the next resident to move in versus the family's need not to feel rushed.
   b. Mary was placed on comfort care. What should be offered to families of those on comfort care? How should their needs be met? In what ways are their ways not being met?
   c. If family needs are not being met, how can that be changed? What would you like to do before or after a death if you had time? What could be done to allow the health care providers to be more effective in such situations?
   d. If you were in the position of a family member and your loved one was on comfort care in a nursing home

or at their own home, what would be your expectations of the staff? Do it area by area, e.g., dietary, nursing, social services, etc.

    e. Would the expectations listed in 1d be met in your community under current practices? If not, what changes have to take place to do so?

2. What are appropriate health care policies and procedures concerning the pending death or death of a resident? How does it vary depending on the facility or staff?

    a. Who is responsible for reviewing the policies and procedures?

    b. Who has the authority to change them?

3. In what ways should health care providers be given closure when a resident dies?

Friends for Life

1. Due to Alfred's declining condition, it was necessary to transfer him from one part of the facility to another. What should be required in the policies and procedures for transfers within a facility? What should be done for the resident to make the transition easier?

2. Thinking of the elderly you know:

    a. Is it important to make sure that every elderly person is able to get away from where they live for a change of scenery? Would that enhance the quality of life for the person?

    b. Should facilities have a policy that requires making sure that residents can go to other parts of the facility and other parts of the community?

    c. If your answer is yes to 2b, the issue often raised is "We don't have enough staff time." If, however, you think it is important for the elderly to have a change of scenery from time to time, how could this be accomplished?

3. The aides and Alfred were in engaged in a situation that called for conflict resolution. How would *you* have handled the situation? Is there conflict-resolution training for caretakers and families of the elderly (not only as they deal with the elderly, but also as they deal with one another)? For that matter, should the elderly be taking conflict-resolution training themselves? Discuss why it would be helpful to receive it.

Always Aim for the Bull's-eye

1. Harold was known as Mr. Public Relations. Are there people in your community who fulfill that function?
    a. If there are such individuals, in what ways might you formally designate them to officially represent your community?
    b. If you had a group of elderly who would serve as public relations people, in what creative ways would you use them? In what ways could you encourage and train those who would like to fulfill that role?
    c. Which elderly are advocates for other elderly? How does the rest of the community, especially health care providers, view these individuals? Are they encouraged, discouraged, listened to, or ignored?
    d. Are health care providers encouraged to be advocates for the elderly? If so, in what ways?

2. Harold said he was an expert on gerontology. Consider the elderly as resource people for seminars, panel discussions, educating your own community, etc. How might you use them?

All wisdom is not taught in your school.

— *Hawaiian Proverb*

Moving On

Have you ever had what you initially thought was just going to be a casual conversation with someone only to have it turn out to be one that you later would reflect upon as being memorable? Memorable not in the sense of simply meeting an unusual personality nor even necessarily hearing memorable stories, but rather, memorable in terms of learning a basic truth to take with you in your journey in life. I had the privilege of having such an experience with a resident by the name of Delbert.

Delbert startled me one morning when he, like a phantom, suddenly appeared at the open door to my office. One moment I had glanced up from the paper work I was doing at my desk and looked out into the hallway at the ramp leading up to the Chronic Care Center — no one was in sight. After leaning back in my chair, rubbing the back of my neck, and stretching out my arms, I returned to my work. I hadn't written more than a sentence or two when I intuitively had the feeling I was no longer alone. I was right. When I looked up, Delbert was standing in my doorway; his head and shoulders were slightly bowed. He was smiling, rather shyly, and his eyes were peering over the rims of his bifocal glasses. Delbert, a very unassuming man who always spoke in a voice barely above a whisper, asked in an apologetically tone of voice, "Can I come in for a rest?"

"Sure, come on in," I replied, actually welcoming the interruption. I figured we would talk for a few minutes and then Delbert would be on his way. Both of us could have a little breather. "Have a chair."

As Delbert and I sat in my office, we chatted about a number of unrelated subjects: the hot humid weather that caused his joints to ache; the baseball game his great-grandson played in last week (they lost 14 to 8); the pair of glasses Delbert misplaced and took an hour to find. "Can't see without them," he said. "How can you look for something when you need glasses in the first place to help you see?" He thought this was humorous and chuckled quite loudly. His laugh in itself was memorable. The only way I can describe his laugh is to say that it sounded like he was blowing up a balloon very rapidly. I'm not sure what proved to be the catalyst, but he began reminiscing about where he grew up. He described the small grain mill his father owned and operated in South Dakota.

"It was originally built as a flour mill in 1864," Delbert said proudly. All the time he was talking, he was peering over his glasses at me. At one point his glasses almost slipped off the edge of his nose. "Yes, sir," he continued as he pushed up his glasses, "it was built by a man who hoped to supply flour to the Northern Army during the Civil War."

"Is that so?" I said, not having known this part of Delbert's history. In the past, he had always been pretty tight-lipped about his family background. Why he was opening up today, I didn't know, but he had my interest. "Tell me more."

"Sure will," he replied as he settled back in his chair. "It seemed like he thought he would be making a lot of money." Delbert chuckled again and I imagined another balloon being blown up. After he caught his breath, he finished his story. "The War ended and the man's dreams for prosperity ended with it." I envisioned a third balloon being blown up when he snickered again. It was quite obvious that he saw some humor in this man's folly.

Delbert went on to tell me that his grandfather purchased the flour mill in 1875 and converted it into a grain mill. He went into detail, describing what had to be done to make the conversion, most of which seemed to me to be quite technical. The grandfather operated the mill until his son, Delbert's father, took it over in 1915. Delbert remembers sitting on the grass in the shade of a tree one summer watching father put a new tin roof on the mill. "I guess I must have been about seven, eight years old at the time." He vividly recalled the first day he began helping at the mill and his father instructing him on how to lift the heavy sacks of grain. "You don't lift with your back," his father warned. "You lift with your knees." Delbert said that he inherited the mill from his father and ran it until the mid 1960s. The day his father turned it over to him was filled with mixed emotions. Delbert was thrilled with the thought of taking it over, but felt sad about seeing his father no longer able to continue to do the work that he so loved to do.

"What ever happened to the mill?" I asked, recognizing how much it had been a part of Delbert's family history.

"Oh, it just sat on the property for years. After I retired, nobody wanted to buy it. I don't blame them." Delbert paused as if waiting for me to ask why. I was just about to do so when he went on. "It was too small an operation and couldn't compete with all the big grain mills. When it didn't sell, we boarded it up."

I wondered if that had been traumatic for him since it had been so much part of his life. "What happened, then?" I asked.

"Over the years it got pretty run down," Delbert replied. "Part of the tin roof my father had put on it was blown off in a storm." He smiled and I wondered what that was about. "Ten, twelve years ago, the whole thing was torn down," he explained, again with a smile. "The foundation's still there. I guess anyone driving by would know that something had been there at one time."

"And how about now?"

"My cousin told me that there's a fence around it." He paused and I knew he wanted me to ask why. When I did, he answered, "Had to keep the kids from playing around that old foundation. Wouldn't want to cause any injuries, would we?" His glasses were slipping to the end of his nose again. "Those things could be dangerous if you're not careful." He pushed up his glasses. "Kids are curious, you know."

I was curious also: How did Delbert feel about no longer having the mill a part of his life? How did it feel to walk away from something that had been such an integral part of his family? How did he feel when it was torn down?

"Was it hard on you when you boarded it up?" I asked, knowing I was probing an area that might be emotional for him. I was prepared for his not wanting to talk about it.

"Oh, no, it was time," he replied in a tone of voice that didn't have the slightest hint of a sense of loss or sadness.

"How about when it was torn down?"

"No, it was getting run down." He tugged at his ear lobe for a moment. "In a few years it probably would have fallen down on its own anyway."

"Were you there when it was torn down?" I asked, again wondering if there was any sense of loss on his part.

"No," he said calmly, "I didn't have a need to, and I haven't seen the spot since they tore it down." He paused for a moment. "I've been told that part of the old wooden fence that ran along side of it was still standing. My cousin said it became part of the new fence they built."

"Really?"

"Yup," he replied with a smile. "That section of the old wooden fence is all that is left; that and the foundation."

Delbert went on to talk about the years after he sold the mill, and the things he and his wife had done. They both came to the nursing home two years ago when his wife suffered a major stroke and was placed in the Chronic Care Center. Although Delbert moved into one of the more independent living areas, he was beginning to physically decline in health as well. He sees his wife two or three times every day. She, however, does not respond to him, and Delbert only hopes she knows he is there when he visits her. It is obvious that he feels lonely without her by his side as he shared several stories how the two of them worked together running the grain mill.

"Oh, that old grain mill has many good memories for me and the Missus. We had a lot of good years there."

Delbert sighed and then looked beyond my open office door into the hallway. He seemed to be revisiting old memories. After a few moments of silence, he said, "That's in the past, though. I have learned that you need to move on with your life."

That the grain mill dated back to the Civil War and had been such an integral part of Delbert's family history was very interesting, but it was not the most memorable aspect of our visit together. What was memorable was his attitude and resolve to face the future, to move on and not look back. For anyone who thinks that the elderly live only in the past, I would like them to meet a man by the name of Delbert.

Move Over Michelangelo

One could call Lyle the Michelangelo of the third floor.

Although Lyle's work perhaps is not equal to the Sistine Chapel, his devotion to his beloved art form would have made Michelangelo proud. Other than going to the dining room for his meals and picking up his mail whenever he was reminded his box was overflowing, Lyle was seldom seen outside his room. He lived on the third floor of the Board and Care section of our facility. Visits to the nurses' station for routine checkups were considered by Lyle to be a nuisance, and the dispensing of his daily medications by the trained medication aides were unwelcome interruptions to his work. He rarely went to resident activities, not because he was unsociable, but rather because he simply was too busy with his art. In his late eighties, Lyle felt he could not afford to waste time.

Visiting Lyle at any time of the day, one no doubt would find him sitting in his swivel chair, hunched over his dark oak desk while working on his beloved projects. He used a variety of items in creating his art: tweezers, an assortment of magnifying glasses, glue, scissors, razor blades, scotch tape, rulers of various lengths, pins, and a few paper clips. Against one wall of his ten by twelve living quarters were stacks upon stacks of various kinds of magazines, newspapers, and posters. In addition to these items, there were dozens of outdated monthly calendars; the years were inconsequential as long as the calendar months had pictures at the top. From this collection of raw materials that staff and friends supplied, Lyle would cut out the pictures, using them to create interesting, beautiful, often intriguing, sometimes puzzling, but always uniquely fascinating collages.

That Lyle and Michelangelo might be considered soul mates

comes from a story about the famous artist. The story is told of Michelangelo that one day he was walking along a quarry and saw a huge block of discarded marble that had been tossed there by another sculptor who felt it was of no value. Michelangelo stopped and studied the piece for quite some time. When asked what he was doing, he replied that he was looking at a beautiful angel.

Lyle would have completely understood the thought process that Michelangelo went through when he saw that block of marble that had been tossed aside. He would have identified with the sculptor's emotions, and he certainly would have understood the passion to create. Lyle, in like manner, saw in those piles of old discarded magazines and outdated calendars the raw materials for the creating of a beautiful piece of art.

Staff would always be welcomed to Lyle's room as long as they were not there to take his blood pressure or to give him medicine. Even when such necessary staff visits were made, however, and after Lyle had put up his usual fuss, he used the opportunity to show them his current work. Very often, Lyle continued to work at his desk during a visit. As he sat, he would swivel his chair back and forth from the desk to the visitor as he talked. Once, a staff member had to take his blood pressure while he was sitting at his desk pondering a critical next step in his work. One of the times I visited him, he pointed out the complexities of putting the pictures together in a way that reflected unity and cohesiveness. His pictures showed a precision in how the various parts related to each other. That was not surprising because Lyle had an engineering background and he loved understanding how an engine fitted together so that all of its various parts contributed to the movement of the whole. Although he never said so, I suspected he was trying to do the same with his collages, positioning the individual pictures within the collage so that each would contribute to the beauty of the whole. He was attempting to combine the precision of engineering with the aesthetic beauty of art.

"Do you see how that fits in there?" he once asked me as I looked at a picture he was just beginning. "You have to get it just right or else it will look like it's just a bunch of pictures pasted together. Do you see that?"

"I think I do, but I'm not sure how all of it will fit together," I said. "Lyle, where do you get your ideas?"

"Oh, I don't know," he replied, peering out at me through thick glasses that made his eyes appear twice as large as they were, "the ideas just come."

On an end table next to his desk was a stack of finished collages, each one carefully separated from another by brown wrapping paper. Back in the corner opposite his desk was a packing carton that his television set came in, but was now filled with all the art work that he had done since first becoming a resident six years ago. His room had become his studio and he took great pleasure in being surrounded by what he had accomplished.

Michelangelo probably does not need to worry about his masterpieces being overshadowed by Lyle's collages, but I can't help believing that the two of them would have a lot to talk about if they should ever happen to meet. Both Michelangelo and Lyle found beauty in the world in which they lived, often in that which others discarded or overlooked.

The Man with Eleven Eyes

"I have eleven eyes," Marshall said to me one afternoon as we sat in his room and talked. Actually, I mainly listened as he expounded ideas and shared insights on life. He covered a wide range of subjects, speaking philosophically upon such things as how the game of baseball has changed over the years, the blessings and curses of growing old, the importance of prayer and spirituality, fishing for bass, talk radio shows, and the Model T Ford he drove as a young man that he claimed was "the best darn car I ever owned."

In his early nineties, Marshall willingly shares his thoughts on most anything, approaching the subject like a modern-day Socrates or Plato. Consider the following sampling of his musings: baseball needs to be played on grass and in the open air because man has to breath and feel the natural elements to realize his oneness with nature; growing old is not for everyone — especially for those who have a difficult time with change; all of us have a spiritual side, and we get into trouble when it is ignored; bass are the only fish worth going after; listening to talk radio when you're blind is like reading a book with your ears; the Model T was one machine a man could fall in love with. "That old Model T could spit like an angry cat, but it sure could purr like a kitten when it had a mind to." He also will tell you that Henry Ford was a genius and should have run for president.

Marshall has been a resident for nearly seven years, living most of those years in the Chronic Care Center. When he first arrived at our facility, his vision was quite poor, but he still managed to pursue his love of reading with the help of a magnifying glass. Unfortunately, within a period of several months, his vision deteriorated until he could no longer see the print, even with a magnifying glass. At his request, his beloved books were given to the resident library. Marshall's eyesight continued to fail with the passage of time. Tables and chairs became blurred objects, while people were indistinguishable shapes only recognizable by voices and movement. Although his thick-lens glasses were no longer of any use, he continued to wear them because, as he said, "They're like an old friend. I've worn them all my life and I'd feel naked without them."

The afternoon we visited, I listened with interest as he shared his wisdom on sports, theology, fishing, and the like. It was during our discussion about the blessings and curses of old age that Marshall made his comment about having eleven eyes. That comment, more than any other, reflected the benevolent approach he has toward life. At first, I didn't know what he meant until he raised his hands, palms up, smiled, and stretched out his fingers. "These are my eyes and I can see many things with them."

I was puzzled. "Marshall, that's only ten," I said. "You told me that you had eleven eyes. Where's the other one?"

Without saying a word, Marshall placed his hand over his heart, and patted his chest a couple of times, looking in my direction and smiling.

Until three years ago, Marshall, using his walker, managed to navigate reasonably well by his count-the-steps-methods.

"It's seven steps to the doorway of my room from this here chair I'm sitting in," he explained as he pointed toward the doorway. "Then, after turning left, it's twenty-eight steps to the first turn in the corridor ..." he paused for a moment. "And another seventy-three steps until I reach a chair at the bottom of the ramp."

"Is that the one that's just around the corner?" I asked, mentally visualizing at what point Marshall was in the trek he was describing.

"Yes, sir, that's the one," he replied. "I stop and rest there, and then gather up my strength to make the final 112 steps to my favorite chair in the lobby; the one with the thick cushions next to the piano."

Since our facility went through a major building and renovation project, however, it hasn't been as easy for Marshall to find his way. "Everything has changed so much," he said, and then added with his characteristic sense of humor, "including me." When Marshall does venture out now, he has to depend upon others whom he meets along the way. He'll stop at any chair to sit until he is able to get the attention of someone walking by. If there are no available chairs, he will stand patiently until someone comes by. Marshall will try to get their attention, but that doesn't always work because as he says, "Some of them are in such a hurry that they don't seem to see me." When he does get someone's attention, he will ask where he is and asks directions to where he wants to go. "I'm one man," he says, "who isn't afraid to stop and ask for directions. I used to do it all the time when I was driving the Model T."

While Marshall never laments his blindness, he does express frustration about those who greet him as they walk by without telling him who they are. "I know many of them by the sound of their voices, but sometimes I get voices confused. It sure would help if they'd say their name each time. They think that just because I wear these here glasses I can see." Marshall also expresses bewilderment about those who walk by without acknowledging his asking for help. "Don't those people know the story of the Good Samaritan?" he asks. "I'm the one who's blind, and yet they walk by as if they can't see me." His biblical reference reflects his life-long attempt to model a help-your-neighbor behavior. This was especially evident two years ago when his roommate was dying. They had become good friends in the three years they shared a room. Walking by their door, I would often hear Marshall leading the two of them in prayer or reciting the Twenty-Third Psalm. When asked about what he did for his friend, he was quite humble. "Oh, I could see he needed some comfort. I did what I could." For Marshall, spirituality is very important, and he would say it has helped him with his blindness. He shared a story about a stay in the hospital when he was in his early seventies that, I think, helps explain who he is. In the hospital, his condition became critical, and he was put on IVs and oxygen.

"I had all kinds of tubes sticking out of me," Marshall said. "Wasn't sure I'd make it. I went into a deep sleep," he paused for a moment, and then sighed. "I suppose they thought I was in a coma or something. During this sleep, I found myself sitting on the banks of the most beautiful lake. Do you know who was with me?"

"No, I don't."

"It was the Lord," he said quietly. "It was so peaceful. Then my sister, Helen, was there. She died of cancer five years earlier. She told me to hang on to the Twenty-Third Psalm. I have ever since. I repeat it every night before I go to bed."

Marshall's health has further declined, and he is too weak now to walk even with the aid of his walker. Consequently, he seldom leaves his room, and when he does, he is taken in a wheelchair. His meals are brought to him, and at times, he has to be fed by a staff person. Even as frail as he is, staff continues to be impressed by how insightful Marshall can be about their lives. One nursing assistant shared how Marshall astonished him one afternoon.

"I was giving Marshall a bath," he said, "and we were just talking about things when he tells me how sorry he is that I have problems with my home life. I asked him, 'How do you know that?'"

"What did he say?" I asked.

The nursing assistant's face took on a look of astonishment as he replied, "The only thing he said was, 'Oh, I can see.'"

I thought to myself, *That eleventh eye really does see many things.*

Crazy is as Crazy Does

"&*/#@*&!" Mathilda was yelling and screaming obscenities again. Her outburst this time was directed at a nurses' aide who was merely trying to do his job. Mathilda was in the lounge area of the main lobby reading a newspaper when the aide approached her to ask if she would return to her room. His request had been made so that he could attend to her medical needs. Mathilda's right foot had a badly infected big toe, and the doctor had left instructions that it was to be soaked in warm water twice a day.

When I happened upon the scene, Mathilda was wildly swinging her arms like a windmill gone berserk. This windmill's fists, however, were clenched, ready to do battle. Although Mathilda was in a wheelchair, and weighed no more than 100 pounds dripping wet, she wanted everyone to know she was no eighty-eight-year-old weakling. Having had other encounters with her, the aide was wisely keeping his distance. He explained to me later why the newspaper was scattered on the floor around her wheelchair; she had thrown it at him.

"Leave me the &*/#@*& hell alone," Mathilda had screamed at him. The words had flown from her like angry hornets whose nest had been disturbed. "Get the &/@* out of here."

The aide looked helplessly at me, raised his eyebrows, and shrugged his shoulders to signal that he didn't know what to do. The expression upon his face told me that he was giving up for the time being. He had already spent fifteen minutes trying to convince Mathilda that what he was asking her to do was for her own good. What he needed to do now was go to the nurses' station and document in the chart about her outburst. After that, I advised him that he should seek support from other staff that have also taken care of her and have been the subject of her outbursts. He told me that he would approach Mathilda again after his afternoon break, but this time he said that the foot soaking could not be put off again. It would have to be done and he would have to do it.

"Well, Mathilda," the aide said in a remarkably calm tone of voice, given the circumstances, "I guess we can do the foot soaking later this afternoon."

"You &*/#@8& damn right you can," Mathilda retorted, giving him a stern look. "That's what I told you in the first place. If you had any blankety-blank sense," she chastised, "you would have listened."

Having said her piece, Mathilda watched triumphantly as the aide walked away. No sooner had he walked out of earshot than she motioned for me to come closer. I walked over and knelt down in front of her.

"They don't think what I'm doing, all that yelling and cussing, is normal," Mathilda said in a voice that she probably thought was no louder than a whisper. Her volume, however, was loud enough that anyone within ten feet could hear. I noticed the woman at the receptionist desk look in our direction and smile. "They probably think I'm off my rocker," Mathilda cried and then pointed to her head. "Perhaps they think I'm a little touched up here because of my age."

"Oh, I'm sorry," I said, trying to be sympathetic.

"No!" she exclaimed. "That's good." She gave a wicked chuckle as a look of victory came over her craggily lined face. "That's exactly what I want them to think — that I'm crazy. Maybe then they'll leave me alone."

Mathilda continues to play her game of acting crazy with staff. One morning another nursing aide who had been at the nursing home less than a week motioned at me as I was walking by. "Will you go see Mathilda?" she asked in a desperate tone of voice. There was a look of fear in her eyes. "I think she may have gone over the edge."

"Sure," I replied, wondering what Mathilda had pulled this time. "I'll go, but why do you think that?"

"I went to tell her that she'll be having a bath soon, and she started screaming and swearing at me." The aide, her voice still trembling, took a deep breath before going on. "She told me that she wasn't going to take any blankety-blank bath until she wanted to. That woman even picked up a hair brush and was going to throw it at me if I didn't get out of her room."

"I suppose, then, you got out?" I asked, figuring that's what I would do. Personally, I would have no desire to be in the same room with an eighty-eight-year-old wildcat, even if she was in a wheelchair.

"I sure as hell did get out," she blurted out, and then got a pained expression on her face. "Oh, I'm sorry, Chaplain. I didn't mean to swear, but that woman ..."

"That's okay," I reassured her. Having overheard the ranting and ravings of Mathilda, I felt there was nothing that anyone else could say that could make me blush. "Go on with your story."

"Thank you," she said, obviously relieved, and then took a deep breath before continuing on with her tale. "I left for a few minutes, thinking she needed some time to cool off. When I came back five minutes later, Mathilda had barricaded herself in her room. I think she had a chair up against the door."

"A chair?" I asked, wondering if there was such a thing as a nursing home SWAT team that could be called in on these situations. "Are you talking about her wheelchair?"

"No, another chair. I saw it when I managed to push the door open a couple of inches. Don't ask me how she did it, but it was there. And then she yelled, 'You're not blankety-blank coming in here!'" The nursing aide took another deep breath. "I tell you, Chaplain," she said, shaking her head, "that woman's absolutely crazy."

I suggested that she go on break and have a cup of coffee or to talk to her supervisor who, I know, has consoled others about Mathilda. I thought about quipping that she might have to wait in line, but I decided not to. After she left, I went to Mathilda's room, took a deep breath, and knocked on the door.

"Mathilda," I said tentatively, not knowing what was going to happen, "it's the Chaplain. May I come in?"

The door opened a crack and Mathilda asked in a voice that she still thought was just a whisper, "Is she gone?"

"She's gone," I replied.

"Does she think I'm crazy?"

I shook my head as I smiled inwardly. "I think you could count on that."

"Good!" she shouted so exuberantly that I thought she might jump out of her wheelchair and dance a jig.

Mathilda has been a resident for nearly eight years, living the last five in the Chronic Care Center. She became a resident shortly after her husband died. Prior to her husband's unexpected death from a massive heart attack, they had lived in their home for nearly sixty years. Two months after he died, she announced to her family that she had made the decision to move to "the place where the old people go." Each of her two daughters offered to have her come live with them but she declined, saying that she had already made her decision. Over the years, she would proudly tell and retell the story to the staff of how she had made up her mind one day that she was moving into a nursing home, and the very next day had informed her daughters at a grandson's birthday party. She told me that she had not sought her family's advice nor asked their opinion. "That way, the decision was made," she explained. "Nobody could argue. They have their own lives to live and are busy with their grandkids. They don't need to have me in the way. I can take care of myself."

Her daughters were actually quite relieved when Mathilda informed them of her decision. They knew her well enough to know that if she had moved in with either of them, they would have had their hands full — not because of the physical care their mother may have needed, but because of her strong will and unyielding determination to live life the way she thought she had the right. Whenever the daughters visited their mother at the Home, they make a point of thanking the staff in Mathilda's presence for taking such good care of their mother. The staff understood what the daughters were saying, smiled knowingly, and accepted their expression of gratitude.

That Mathilda was strong willed and, at times, unreasonable was something both her family and the staff agreed upon. In fairness, however, she should not have always been viewed in such an unfavorable light. There were occasions when, looking at the situation from her perspective, you might agree that she did have valid reasons for her actions. One example of how her actions were unfairly characterized as being unreasonable was when she told me how she declined her oldest daughter's invitation to spend a couple of days at her house over the Thanksgiving Day holiday.

"The great-grandchildren will be there and they'd love to have you stay," the daughter had said to Mathilda, trying to persuade her mother to change her mind. "You'll have your own bedroom, you can go to bed at any time, and sleep as late as you want. We can pick you up on Thursday morning and take you home on Saturday."

The daughter, after her mother had said no for a second time, knew her mother's temperament well enough not to pursue the matter any further. Why her mother would rather go back to her room at the Home instead of spending time with family members was something that Mathilda's daughter felt had no reasonable explanation. When Thanksgiving arrived, Mathilda did spend part of the day with her daughter and the great-grandchildren, but had requested to be brought back to the nursing home before it got dark.

"I love my great-grandchildren but one day with them is enough," Mathilda told me during a visit I had with her the week following Thanksgiving. "It's just too much activity and noise. Then there's my hearing; it has gotten to the point that I don't like being in a group where people are talking all at once. It sounds like a lot of mumbo-jumbo to me." Mathilda also shared that she worried about the weather. "I might not have gotten back in time if the weather was bad. It seems like it always snows on Thanksgiving. Then I would worry about them driving back in it." She also went on to tell me that she didn't want to stay overnight because she was more comfortable in her own bathroom, her own bed, and having her own nightly routine. When I asked if she had explained this to her daughter, Mathilda shook her head and said no; she didn't think her daughter would understand.

"When you have a bladder problem and have to get up in the middle of the night, you don't want an unfamiliar bathroom," Mathilda said. "I don't think my daughter will completely understand until she gets to be my age and has a few plumbing problems of her own."

When the nursing aide located Mathilda later that afternoon and asked her to come back to her room so that her foot could be soaked, I heard that she threw a shoe at him and yelled, "Where the &*/#@*& have you been? My foot's hurting. It should've been taken care of this morning. Just you wait till the doctor hears about this."

The poor guy went away muttering out loud to anyone who would listen, "That woman is crazy!"

Actions Speak Louder than Words

In his early nineties, Sid is an individual who could very well serve as a role model for the younger generation. I know that after spending some time with him, they would come away saying, "That old guy is as sharp as a tack. I hope I can be like that when I'm his age."

Besides being sharp as a tack, Sid also cares deeply about people. However, one might not always discover that in conversations with him simply because engaging him in a conversation is seldom easy. It certainly isn't because he's unfriendly, or shy, or simply unable to converse. Quite the contrary; he is very pleasant to be with and, as I have already mentioned, very knowledgeable. If he wanted to, he could carry on a discussion with just about anyone on almost any subject.

The reason that having a conversation with Sid is difficult is quite simple — he is a man of such few words. One would not get to know him very quickly because he mainly listens, only responding to questions when asked. His answers are brief, yet always to the point, and spoken with a keen awareness of the subject being discussed. He will acknowledge your statements with a nodding of the head or raising of his eyebrows, but he seldom offers his thoughts or insights about the subject unless he is asked. He is one of the most unassuming individuals you will ever meet.

Sid seldom talks about or shows his feelings, and one could mistakenly think he is simply a private person who prefers to keep to himself. One might even wonder about the claim that he is a man who deeply cares about others. On the surface, this may seem to be the case, but only on the surface. As one begins to know and understand Sid, one discovers that he expresses his feelings and emotions in non-verbal ways.

Like many in his generation, Sid grew up in an era when individuals lived by the motto, *Actions speak louder than words.* To get a measure of his compassion for others, therefore, one needs to see him in action. The prime example of how Sid lives this motto is seen whenever he sits down at a piano. On such occasions the keyboard becomes an extension of him and it is here that one understands how this man of few words demonstrates his caring for others. It is through his playing that Sid touches the lives of others in ways that words cannot adequately express. Twice a week he takes his place at the grand piano in the main lobby of our facility. The lobby, known as Heritage Hall, dates back to the early days when there was only one building called The Lodge. The lobby itself is often compared to a lobby one might expect to find when visiting some historic grand old hotel: rich, dark oak paneling; beautiful floral design carpeting; an elegant fireplace; floor to ceiling dark oak pillars; comfortable sofas and matching chairs; beautiful ornate lamps; and vases of fresh flowers all make the lobby a very inviting place to sit, play a friendly game of cards, or to listen to those who come in to play the piano.

As Sid's hands glide across the keyboard, the residents who have gathered to listen and enjoy his music settle back in their chairs. If one were to walk through the lobby during this time, one would see the joy on their faces as Sid brings back memories with his renditions of the "good old songs." He knows he is touching their hearts with their kind of music, and they know that he cares for them by playing it. Most of the residents sit quietly. Here and there are those who drum their fingers against the soft padded arm of their chairs; a few tap their feet in rhythm. Depending on the song, a half dozen or so will sing, perhaps off key, but no one notices nor cares. Every now and then, a resident will ask another to dance. On this day, a husband and wife hold hands as they sit in their wheelchairs, glancing at each other every now and then, silently listening to music that rekindled memories of years gone by.

Sid characteristically says very little to those gathered. He silently comes in, takes his place at the piano, and without any sheet music, begins to play. After a half hour to forty-five minutes, he stands, nods his head ever so slightly to acknowledge the applause, and leaves. A quiet man, Sid lets the music speak for him; it is his way of making a contribution to the lives of others. His playing the piano shows them he cares.

Sid and others of his age grew up believing that they had a moral obligation to give something of themselves to the world in which they were born. Many of his generation saw responsibility as a privilege. They may have agonized over the number of deaths brought on by World War I, partied through the Roaring Twenties, stood in soup lines during the Great Depression, survived the heartache of World War II, but through it all, and because of such experiences, they made the commitment to leave the world a little bit better off. Sid and his peers try to live as an example to others. Words like honesty, integrity, honor, loyalty, and commitment meant something to them and still do; that is the reason everyone knows that on certain days of the week at the appointed hour, an unassuming man will walk in to fulfill what he has agreed to do. There are no signed agreements, for none are needed. For Sid and those like him, to give your word is good enough; a handshake would be accepted without question as a promise that would be kept.

Sid's wife died last year on the day of their sixty-third wedding anniversary. The next day, he and I sat in his room sharing the moment and unspoken feelings, engaging in little conversation. When he did speak, it was about finalizing the necessary funeral arrangements. His wife's death was ironic because she had been more concerned about his medical problems than her own. Their marriage had been built on selfless devotion and love for each other. She once told me that Sid had always been a loving and devoted husband, and that she felt lucky to have married him. When she died, Sid quietly grieved for his wife in his own way, but he confided in me that he had been lucky to find such a wonderful woman.

The next day I was told that Sid was playing the piano for the other residents. I overheard several staff and residents speak in admiration of how this man could do this having lost his wife just two days before. I think the answer as to how he could do it came in the music he shared. The first tune he played was *It Had To Be You ... Wonderful You*. His final number for the afternoon's concert spoke volumes as he played *I'll Be Loving You Always*.

While remembering his wife, Sid was still giving to others. Once again, this man of few words was living by the motto — Actions speak louder than words.

Questions for Reflection

These questions are meant to be catalysts, to stimulate creative thinking about ways at providing quality, holistic care for the elderly. In some instances, the reflecting may lead to new (perhaps untraditional) ways of providing care. Not all questions may apply to your situation, but *all* situations will benefit from reflecting upon them. Whether your community is a long-term care facility, a new retirement home, or the old neighborhood, you can adapt them to fit your situation.

Moving On

1. Recognizing the health benefits of laughter and humor, in what ways does your community promote laughter and humor for *all* those who live and work there?
    a. Take a walk through your community, both meeting places and living areas: do you see smiles on the faces of the elderly and hear laughter? Discuss your observations.
    b. Do another walk through your community, and this time pay attention to the people working there. Do they seem happy and joyful? Do you see smiles and hear laughter? Share your observations and discuss what you have observed.
    c. Reflect how your community could be a happier (and healthier) environment for both the elderly and their caretakers.

2. Discuss the value to caretakers and the elderly of having a seminar on the therapeutic benefits of humor. In what ways might both benefit if you had this seminar?

3. One of the benefits of having a happy environment is that it reduces stress among those who live or work in it. With that in mind:
    a. Name and discuss the three major stressors in your community.
    b. How do you feel that those stressors in 3a could be reduced?

4. Is your community committed to reducing stress for caretakers? If so, how is that commitment shown in concrete ways? List them and discuss their effectiveness.
    a. If your community decided to commit itself to making a conscious effort at reducing stress for caretakers, what would be the first steps in doing so?

    b. How do you feel about the statement, "Stress for caretakers can be reduced only when the whole community commits itself to it."? In a facility this would mean commitment from the top down as part of its corporate culture.

    c. Envision a "Stress-Reduction Task Force." What would be its statement of purpose? Goals? Who would serve on it?

    d. What can *you* do to reduce stress for others? (List all the other people who are impacted by what you do, and then ask yourself: How are other people affected if I do not do my job well? How does doing my job poorly add stress to other people?)

    e. Discuss innovative ways for reducing stress among caretakers (for example, engaging the services of a professional masseuse for a day to provide massages).

5. Delbert talked about the losses in his life. Do the caretakers in your community have the training to understand the many losses a person experiences when they grow older, including the losses caused by moving into a nursing home?

6. Caretakers can also suffer losses. For example, those who are taking care of family members suffer a loss each time the person they are caring for suffers a loss.

    a. Discuss how personal losses for caretakers affect their level of care giving.

    b. Discuss how caretakers' stress affects their level of care giving.

Move Over Michelangelo

1. In what ways does your community promote and/or encourage resident hobbies and interests? Brainstorm things that could be tried that haven't been tried before.

2. Lyle's hobby involved creating beauty out of the ordinary things in life. Do a tour of your community and then discuss:
   a. Would you describe the care your elderly receive as "institutional"? Why or why not? What parts of it are more institutional than others?
   b. What objects of *beauty* do you see in your part of the community that contribute to a feeling of its being non-institutional?
   c. How could you beautify areas (including the institutional areas) within your community?
   d. Discuss the implications for resident care of the following: Do caretakers work in someone's home or do the elderly live in someone's place of work?

3. What kinds of things would the elderly like to see within their environment? Do a survey. Write down *everything* suggested and be open to making changes.

4. If you were a resident in a facility, what would be important for you to see as part of your environment?

5. How could areas for caretakers (where they eat, take breaks, etc.) be esthetically improved? Ask the caretakers you know what they would like to see for their areas. Be careful about not letting the bottom line (money) stifle your brainstorming.

The Man with Eleven Eyes

1. Marshall wanted staff to say their names when they greeted him. What is the practice of caretakers you know in greeting those they know to be visually impaired?
   a. What kind of message is given to a person when a caretaker assumes the person will recognize her/his voice?
   b. Marshall also talked about staff that pass him by without asking if he needed help. Do you think this is a problem in your community? Why or why not?

    c. How important is it for caretakers in a facility to know the names of all the residents? In what ways can you encourage them to learn the names?

2. Marshall talked about his roommate who was dying:
   a. What special attention should be given to the person who is living with someone who is dying? Think of yourself in that situation — what would be your concerns?
   b. If a resident in a facility does not wish to remain in the room when his/her roommate is dying, should s/he be allowed to move to a different room? Are such temporary rooms available? Should they be? Discuss.
   c. Discuss the concept of providing hospice rooms or facilities (places set aside specifically for residents who are dying).

Crazy is as Crazy Does

1. How should caretakers be trained to handle an elderly person who yells and shouts obscenities?

2. Mathilda's outward behavior (screaming, cussing, etc.) had ulterior motives (wanting to be left alone). In what ways are caretakers trained in discerning residents' ulterior motives? How would this benefit staff in providing daily care?

Actions Speak Louder than Words

1. Sid often expressed himself in non-verbal ways. Since many residents do that:
   a. Are caretakers given training to learn how to read non-verbal communication?
   b. Discuss the many ways caretakers give non-verbal communication (good and bad) to the elderly, families, *and* to other staff.

2. Sid showed his caring for others by playing the piano. In what intentional ways does your community nurture the concept of the elderly caring for other elderly (as well as caring for staff)? What jobs can the elderly do to help others?

Every path has a puddle.

— *English Proverb*

The Tarnished Silver Frame

"Take me home," Mae pleaded as I was leaving the nursing home late one afternoon. She was standing in the entryway looking out the glass doors toward the service road in front of the building. She would first look in one direction and then in the other, her head moving back and forth as if she were watching a tennis match being played in slow motion. When asked whom she was waiting for, she replied, hesitantly, "Oh, I don't remember, but I know somebody is supposed to come." She did not know who was coming, or when they would come. All Mae knew for certain was that she wanted to go home.

Cradled in Mae's arms was an assortment of items: a couple of small picture frames displaying faded black and white photographs, a spiral notebook, a small clock — its cord hanging down to her feet, a hand mirror, two combs, a hairbrush, and several magazines. She had no suitcases or overnight bags. Although the temperature was chilly, Mae was wearing only a short-sleeved blouse and light slacks.

The receptionist and I looked at each other as if to say, what are we going to do? The receptionist later told me that Mae had been standing at the doorway for almost an hour and had declined to sit down when offered a chair. She also said that whenever a car pulled up, Mae pressed herself against the door, anticipating that whoever was in the car had come for her. The smile on Mae's face, however, always faded as the car drove away. She would look at the receptionist and say, "They'll come. I know they will." As the receptionist told me later, "I just smiled in return and nodded. I knew that I didn't need to do anything about Mae unless the poor woman decided to leave the building. I wouldn't have let her go out in the cold dressed the way she was."

In the nearly six months Mae has lived at the nursing home, the sad fact is that nobody has ever come for her. She moved in after a cousin convinced her that she could no longer live alone. The cousin had told the staff that she had visited Mae in her apartment and, on two occasions, found her wearing clothes that looked as if they had been slept in. She also said that she found food in the refrigerator that had spoiled, and a bathroom that appeared as if it had not been cleaned in weeks. The cousin finally knew something had to be done after she stopped one afternoon to visit Mae and discovered that the back burner of the electric stove was on. When she asked about it, Mae could not even remember turning it on. The cousin, herself finding it more difficult to get around because of her own aging, and knowing that she was practically all the family Mae had, decided that Mae had to be in a place where others could watch out for her. The cousin, nearly in tears, had told the staff that she could no longer look out for Mae.

From the first day Mae arrived at the Home, she was found to be a gentle, friendly person with an outgoing personality. In their intake evaluation, the staff determined that she was in reasonably good health and, therefore, would not require a great deal of skilled nursing care. On the basis of that evaluation, Mae was able to move into the independent living section of the facility. Staff were confident that if Mae's basic needs were met — meals in the dining room, daily housekeeping, laundry done for her once a week, and assistance to make sure she wore clean clothing every day — she could live independently. The staff also knew that the more alert residents would help her as they have helped others. They would take Mae to meals with them, help her find her room at those times she became too disoriented, look in on her from time to time, invite her to activities, and so forth.

Everything went fine for the first few months. As time went on, however, it became obvious to both staff and other residents that Mae was becoming more confused, especially in her thinking that her husband would come any day to take her home. Although Mae would be told one day that her husband had died eight years ago, the very next day she would inform people that she would be leaving soon to go home because her husband was coming to get her. Mae had stood waiting at the entryway door before, but according to the receptionist, this was the first time she had brought her "stuff" with her. It was also the first time she had not remembered who was coming to get her.

"Where are you going, Mae?" I asked.

"Why, I'm going home," Mae said in a tone meant to give me the impression that she thought my question was rather strange.

"Mae, you are home," I said quietly. "This is your home."

"It is?" The expression upon her face was a mixture of confusion, surprise, and fear. "I live here?" She glanced around. "Where?"

"You have a nice room on the second floor in the Board and Care building," I replied.

"I do?"

Just at that moment, a housekeeper who worked in Mae's building walked by. The housekeeper, well aware of Mae's increasing dementia, smiled at her, and then said to me, "I'll take her back." After I nodded my appreciation, the housekeeper turned to Mae, "We're friends, aren't we, Mae?" As she walked away with the housekeeper, she could be heard asking, "How long have I lived here?"

That evening, Mae wasn't in her room when another resident came to take her to the dining room. After conducting a search, staff found her walking outside. The temperature had turned quite cold and a light rain was falling. Mae was wearing the same short-sleeved blouse and light slacks. Her lips were blue from the cold, and she was shivering. The only item she was carrying was a faded black and white photograph in a tarnished silver picture frame. The photograph showed a handsome young man sitting in a wooden high-back chair; a beautiful young woman was standing next to him, her right hand on his left shoulder. Mae told the nurse who found her that this was a nice neighborhood. "I don't recognize any of the houses," Mae said, looking up and down the street, "but I'm certain my home is near by." The next day Mae was transferred to the Alzheimer's Care Center.

It has been nearly a year since Mae was transferred. It was, of course, for her own protection. The Alzheimer's Care Center is secure; the doors have a keypad and only those knowing the code (staff or visitors) can enter or leave. For Mae, it was difficult at first, but her dementia has now progressed to the point where she no longer talks about going home.

If you were to visit the nursing home, you might recognize Mae; she's the woman clutching a tarnished silver frame.

Who Cares about Dancing Angels

During the Middle Ages it has been said, though never substantiated by written documents, that one of the questions that those in certain theological circles wrestled with was "How many angels could dance on the head of a pin?" If there was ever such a query, it probably was put forth, tongue-in-cheek, by common folks to the scholastic religious community who they felt were spending too much time pondering questions that had no bearing on everyday life. If Gunda, a resident who has a room on the second floor of the Chronic Care Center, had been around at that time, she would have answered the question (whether it had been asked tongue-in-cheek, or otherwise) quite bluntly: Who cares?

Gunda and her peers at the nursing home are not interested in dealing with ethereal inquiries such as dancing angels, nor do they have the time. They ponder more concrete, immediate concerns: *How soon do I get to lie down? How much longer is it until supper? When can I have another pain pill? Will we have raisin toast tomorrow? When are they going to answer my call light? Have they fixed my dentures yet?* These questions reflect the down-to-earth concerns of residents and are always asked with an awareness of how quickly time is passing. Residents, like Gunda, realize they have reached a point in life where their remaining days can no longer with certainty be measured in years or even months. One resident, for example, who was celebrating his ninety-first birthday, shared his perspective of time with those gathered for the occasion. "I've come to the point in life where my future is now behind me," he said, and then added with a laugh, "Let's hurry up, and cut the cake while I still have time to eat it."

As the clock ticks away, many residents will talk about not having enough time in the day to do all the things they want to do. Their days are filled with such things as crocheting mittens for their great-grandchildren, or answering all the mail they receive from family and friends, or sharing a cup of coffee with the newly acquired friends they have made since arriving at the nursing home. To view time from the perspective of residents, as well as experience their sense of urgency about time remaining, you only need to place yourself in the daily routine of a resident for a week or two. If you did, you would discover your days filled with such time-consuming things as going to physical and occupational therapy, having doctor and dental appointments, conferring with staff about baths and changes in medication. Besides these "necessities" of nursing home life, residents seek to find time to read, attend activities that are of interest to them, participate in outings, (going out to eat, for example, is always a treat but can take an entire afternoon), answer correspondence, entertain visitors, volunteer, serve on resident committees, and take naps (as people half their age, upon finding their days so busy, would need to do as well). One cannot assume that the residents have little to do but watch the hands of the clock while they rock in their rocking chairs. If some residents do watch a clock, it may mean that they are simply making sure they will be on time for whatever activity or appointment they have next on their daily agenda.

People who live in nursing homes have learned to literally take life one day at a time. If they do glance at the clock, it is usually because they want to make sure that old Father Time is giving them sixty minutes to every hour. Consider Edwin, for example. He had just returned from spending eleven days at the hospital. Two years shy of being ninety, he had been in for a rather serious viral infection. For a while, it looked as though he wasn't going to make it. The doctors were not optimistic and even told the family one afternoon that they should plan to spend the night. Edwin, however, to everyone's surprise, did recover. Shortly after he returned from the hospital, I went to visit him in his room in the Chronic Care Center. He was propped up in bed doing a crossword puzzle. As he looked to see who was coming in, his glasses slid to the tip of his nose and nearly fell off. Edwin grinned as he pushed them back up.

"Hello," I said, "how're you doing?" I took note how tired he looked. His hospital stay had aged him.

"Got a tune-up at the hospital," he replied more cheerfully than I had expected. After marking the page of his crossword puzzle book, Edwin set it on the nightstand, muttering to it, "I'll get to you later." He pushed up his glasses, which had slipped again, and then looked me straight in the eye as he announced gleefully, "I'm good for another thirty days!"

Some might hear Edwin's remark as no more than a humorous response, but given his recent experience in the hospital, we both understood that underlying his words was the awareness of time rushing by and how fragile life can be. What he did not say, but was evident by the determined look in his eyes, was that of those thirty days, he was going to make every day count. Knowing Edwin, at the end of that period, he would then say to Father Time, *Let's go for another thirty!*

Another example that illustrates that time is viewed from a different perspective by a nursing home resident comes from my initial encounter with Irma. Before fully assuming my position as chaplain at the Home, it was necessary to honor some commitments in the parish I was still serving. My plan was to work for a week in my new position to get oriented, and then go back to my church to finish up the loose ends. On the last day of that first week on the job, during the noon meal for the residents, I went around to each of the tables to explain my work situation. Irma was sitting at one of the tables, and after she heard me say I would be back in two weeks, she said matter-of-factly, but with a twinkle in her eyes, "I hope I'm still around." It was only later that afternoon that I realized Irma was serious. She hoped to see me in two weeks, but at age eighty-four, Irma could not make any promises. As I was to learn from Irma and other residents, their perspective of time is far different from those of the younger generation.

As stated earlier, residents have neither the time nor the inclination to wrestle with such a question as, how many angels could dance on the head of a pin? There is, though, a question that would make a worthy opponent for those living within any period of history. The question was asked by Gunda, who has been a resident at the Home for nearly twelve years. Other than using a walker and, as Gunda says, *doctoring* with her eyes because of cataracts, she was doing reasonably well for being in her late eighties. That was until she suffered a stroke. For five months, Gunda was involved with physical therapy twice a week, occupational therapy once a week, and speech therapy three times a week. During this time, she regained a good share of her speech, but did not regain the use of her right arm, nor her ability to walk without falling. The physical therapy Gunda had received helped but only to a limited extent. Any further walking she would do would now have to be done with the assistance of staff. At her last care conference, she was informed that she had probably regained as much use of her right arm as she could expect. As far as walking again without assistance, the therapists said they would continue to work with her; but, for now, she would need to use a wheelchair until there were further signs of improvement. Faced with her circumstances, Gunda's question was: "If God can perform miracles, why doesn't He perform one on me?"

I don't know about you, but I think I'd rather deal with the question concerning the dancing angels on the head of the pin.

The Sandwiched Generation

"Oh my, I just don't know what I'm going to do," Ruby said as she searched for answers in the faces of the others sitting around the beautiful, highly polished oak conference table. Ruby, a thin, eighty-three-year-old woman sat timidly in the high-back wooden chair, wringing her hands. "I don't know what I'm going to do," she repeated, momentarily forgetting that her husband, Gilmore, was also in the room and was the reason the meeting had been called. He remained quiet, looking at his wife with searching eyes.

It was obvious to all that he knew his wife was upset, but he couldn't understand why.

Ruby, with Gilmore sitting next to her, had just been informed during the specially called care conference that he would be transferred to the Alzheimer's Care Center within a few days. The move would take place as soon as his room was ready. Even though living with Gilmore the past two years in the Board and Care section of the nursing home had been very difficult for Ruby, she felt the separation from her husband would be worse.

Staff had initially suggested that it might be better if Gilmore didn't attend the care conference because of their concern that the decision, and any discussion following it, could upset him. Ruby, however, didn't agree and had quietly insisted that her husband be included. In a very deliberate but polite manner, Ruby told the staff person who had arranged for the meeting that Gilmore had every right to be there. Furthermore, as Ruby explained with words brimming with raw emotion, she felt that her husband *ought to be* there because throughout their married life, she and Gilmore had always shared the good and bad times together. As far as she was concerned, that had always been the essence of their married life. "If this had been the other way around," Ruby told the staff, "Gilmore would have wanted me here, and for the same reason."

Ruby told me later that she knew that Gilmore didn't comprehend most of what was being discussed at the care conference, but that he had instinctively sensed something was upsetting her, and had placed his hand upon hers. Although Gilmore had a smile, Ruby said that she knew it was not natural, and that the look in his eyes was one she had seen many times in the past year — fear. "I just patted his hand and smiled to reassure him that I was okay." She went on to tell me, however, that her whole body ached with sadness. She felt as if she weighed thousands of pounds and could not have gotten up from her chair even if she had wanted. "I was also afraid that my chair would collapse at any moment from the heavy load I'd been carrying around the past twelve months."

It had been almost a year ago to the day of the care conference that Ruby first noticed that Gilmore was not quite himself. If she had been asked at the time in what way her husband was different, Ruby would have answered that he just seemed to be getting a little more forgetful. From the time she first noticed the changes, Gilmore's behavior became increasingly more strange, and at times, bizarre.

At the care conference, Ruby told the staff that looking at how her husband was behaving now, she wondered if he had mysteriously been whisked away and another man put in his place. The whole experience, which was rapidly turning into a nightmare, culminated in an incident two weeks earlier when Ruby had to call for staff assistance. She became frightened when Gilmore had not recognized her when she returned to their room after having coffee with a friend down the hall. He had demanded that someone get this *strange woman* out of his room or he would call his wife. She became even more fearful when he had made a threatening gesture toward her. At the suggestion of the staff, Ruby left while the social worker and a nurse talked to Gilmore to calm him down. Within an hour (though it seemed like five), Ruby came back and, after knocking, cautiously entered the room. She wasn't sure what to expect. The social worker had advised if Gilmore didn't recognize her, she should just excuse herself, saying that she had the wrong room.

As Ruby entered, Gilmore was sitting in his favorite chair. When he heard the door open, he looked up from the magazine he was reading and asked where she had been; he had missed her. After the same scenario repeated itself two days later, the staff decided that for Ruby's own protection, Gilmore needed to be transferred.

Because of Gilmore's increasing erratic behavior, his short-term memory loss, and other signs of dementia, the whole situation was becoming too taxing on Ruby. The nurses were concerned about her physical and emotional well being. The staff also were concerned that Gilmore could become violent if too agitated. Ruby, for her part, had realized something had to be done, but she always hoped in her heart that Gilmore's condition might improve, and their lives could get back to *normal*. After the care conference, she knew that the word normal would no longer describe her life, as she realized the staff's decision was final. Deep within her, Ruby said she felt such an emptiness that she grieved the loss of all the familiar things about Gilmore she loved; waking up beside him; watching him doze in his chair; being amused by the habits he had learned from his grandfather, like pouring hot coffee into the cup's saucer to sip it; and listening to classical music together. Ruby may have agreed with the staff that it would be best for Gilmore to move, but she asked me if she would ever get over her feelings of emptiness and loss.

You may have heard the expression, "The Sandwiched Generation." The phrase is used to describe those who are caught between dealing with, on the one hand, aging parents and all the problems that can entail while, on the other hand, faced with problems brought on by teenage or adult children. Caught in the middle, those of the sandwiched generation are often stressed-out, emotionally exhausted, and physically drained as they find themselves running from kid problems at school to parent problems at the nursing home. One woman in her forties shared with me that within a period of six months, she had an adult child go through a divorce, a teenager who wanted to quit school, and a mother who called her every day at work from the nursing home, demanding to know why her daughter put her in such a terrible place. In tears, the woman confessed to me, "I can't help it. I just feel like running away from home. I feel angry and sad at the same time."

It may come as a surprise to some, but those who are residents in nursing homes can also qualify for membership in the sandwiched generation. They may not be wedged between the problems of loved ones in the generations ahead and behind them, but they certainly know what it is like to be caught up in the problems of those they love.

Ruby became a member of the sandwiched generation the same week she and Gilmore attended the care conference where she learned of the decision to transfer him to the Alzheimer's Care Center. Besides feeling the sadness of knowing she soon would be living apart from her husband for the first time in fifty-three years and dealing with the grief associated with that, Ruby also had a son who was having major health problems. The son, at sixty-three, had just been told by doctors that he needed bypass surgery. Ironically, the day he called his mother to tell her was the day before the care conference. Ruby's son was aware of the meeting concerning his father and had agonized over whether to call with his news. He knew, however, that he had little choice since surgery had been scheduled within a week, and it would have been worse for his mother if she did not receive the daily phone calls she expected.

Ruby, of course, was upset about her son's news but she was also glad that he told her. Like any mother, Ruby did and continues to worry about her son's health even though the doctors announced that the surgery was a success. "You never cease to be a parent," she said. Ruby and others her age would tell you that the contract for being a parent has no retirement clause.

Sandwiched between her husband's and son's problems, Ruby felt as though she couldn't turn to either one for the support she needed; her husband wasn't able to give it, and she didn't want to put any added pressure upon her son. I think Ruby's situation more than qualifies her for membership in the sandwiched generation.

By the way, in case you are wondering, Ruby's membership in the sandwiched generation is not out of the ordinary. There are many other people who could easily qualify for membership as well: Andrew, age seventy-four; Maxine, age ninety-two; Stuart, age eighty-three …

The Car's in the Garage

"What's the weather like?"

Daisy asks that question six or seven times a day as she sits in her favorite chair in the lounge of the main lobby. She sips lukewarm coffee out of a Styrofoam cup and nibbles on a peanut butter cookie as she eyes the people coming in and out. Her walker, parked along side the chair, is within easy reach in case, as she jokes, "My old bladder begins to act up, and I gotta move fast." As for the answer to her question, it doesn't matter what kind of weather report is given by the person responding to her because Daisy's reply is always the same, "Guess I better leave the car in the garage and stay in. Don't you think?"

As you may have guessed, there is no garage nor is there a car. At age ninety-eight, Daisy's only means of transportation is walking with the aid of her walker. Though she is suffering from short-term memory loss, Daisy is alert enough to understand she is dealing with one of the most difficult losses one can experience: the loss of independence. She sums up her feelings toward that loss quite aptly as far as she is concerned, "It's hell to get old!"

The "car in the garage" Daisy constantly refers to is symbolic of the losses that she and her peers experience. Having a "set of wheels," for example, is just as important for the older generation, and for the same reason, as it is for the younger generation. Perhaps that is why those at the opposite ends of the age spectrum seem to understand each other, at least when it comes to needing the kind of independence that a vehicle provides. Consider the following story as an illustrious example of the common ground that the young and the old can share at times.

> *A teenage grandson told his grandmother that he had to be driven to the nursing home to see her. "Why?" she asked. She knew that he had had his license for over a year. "Because," he said, "I gave some lip to mom over some homework she wanted me to finish, and I wanted to go out with the guys." His grandmother asked what happened, and was told that he had been grounded for a week from driving the car. The grandmother replied that she knew exactly how he felt about being grounded, but then added not to worry; at least, he could drive once the week is up. As for herself, she was grounded for life. "Wow," the grandson replied, looking at her with new respect and a twinkle in his eye, "Grandma, who did you give lip to?"*

Loss of independence for the elderly can be gradual, and when it is, it provides smoother sailing into the potentially turbulent waters of one's later years. The loss, however, can also come at such an alarming speed that one just hangs on for dear life, feeling as if he or she were shooting the rapids toward a roaring waterfall. One woman who recently became a resident shared her experience. "There I was living carefree and independently in my apartment. I thought I was doing pretty good for an old lady. I'm eighty-seven. And then it happened. I was just reaching to put something away on a top shelf, lost my balance, fell, and fractured my hip. In those few seconds, my whole way of life changed."

Concerning this matter of independence, it certainly is far more extensive than just the loss of a car. A person's independence can be chipped away at from many different angles. Family, friends, and even professional caregivers themselves must be careful not to contribute unknowingly to the many ways the elderly can have their independence diminished.

One day I was walking past Leo's room in the Chronic Care Center and for some reason just happened to look in. Leo was in his wheelchair at the foot of his bed, and by the expression on his face I could tell something wasn't right. He looked as if he was in agony and I was concerned that he was possibly having a stroke. Rushing in, I went up to his wheelchair and knelt before him. Since the television was blaring, I yelled, "Leo, are you okay?"

"Can you do something for me?" he moaned.

"I'll do what I can." I was expecting him to ask me to put him into bed, or to get him some pain pills, or call for the nurse.

"Would you turn off the TV?" he pleaded.

"Sure."

The television was tuned to some daytime soap opera in which the actors were involved in a shouting match about someone's husband sleeping with someone else's wife. The volume was so loud, the room sounded like an echo chamber as the sound bounced off the walls. It reminded me of the time I went to a rock concert and got so close to the stage that my chest bones felt as if they were vibrating in sync with the loud speakers. I pushed the button on the TV, and the room got peacefully quiet.

"Oh, thank God, what a relief," Leo muttered as he rubbed his forehead with the palms of his hands and then moved his hands back across his head and down his neck. "That thing was driving me crazy."

Leo told me that someone, he wasn't sure who, turned the television on while he was looking out the window. The person apparently thought he was lonely and needed some company. The television was switched on and the volume turned up. Leo was unable to reach the controls, and was trapped with company he didn't ask for nor want. His independence had been taken away from him on several counts: he wasn't asked if he wanted the set on; once it had been turned on, he wasn't asked which station he wanted to watch; and he wasn't asked about the volume. As to this latter point, Leo was simply the victim of the assumption that all elderly people are hard of hearing.

Independence is as important to people like Daisy and Leo as it would be to any of us. They and their peers recognize that there are aspects of being independent that certainly will succumb to the aging process and the physical limitations that come with it. Living in a nursing home and being dependent upon others is difficult enough, but what can make it even harder are the actions of others who unthinkingly diminish their sense of independence still further.

It is true that both Daisy and Leo no longer enjoy the independence they once had. Nevertheless, there are other areas of their lives over which they can exercise some control and thus feel as if they still can retain some of their independence.

When Daisy talks about leaving the car in the garage, or when we see a tortured look on Leo's face, we should be careful about simply dismissing these things as "things you see and hear when you visit those in a nursing home." Both Daisy and Leo, in their own way, are reminding us of the importance of independence. Consider: Are they asking us to give them back the independence that the aging process has taken away from them, or are they simply asking us to be sensitive enough so that we do not take away what little independence they may have left? It is a question to reflect upon before making that next visit to someone in a nursing home. If you need some advice, you could always talk to Daisy. She is the one nibbling a peanut butter cookie just inside the entrance. Don't worry about intruding upon her. She has plenty of time to talk. She has no plans; she isn't going anywhere. Her car is in the garage.

Questions for Reflection

These questions are meant to be catalysts, to stimulate creative thinking about ways at providing quality, holistic care for the elderly. In some instances, the reflecting may lead to new (perhaps untraditional) ways of providing care. Not all questions may apply to your situation, but *all* situations will benefit from reflecting upon them. Whether your community is a long-term care facility, a new retirement home, or the old neighborhood, you can adapt them to fit your situation.

The Tarnished Silver Frame

1. Mae's cousin convinced Mae to move into a nursing home when she became concerned that Mae could no longer safely take care of herself. What sorts of alternatives for care are available in your community? At what point is it appropriate for a person to move into a more structured care situation?

2. Discuss whether the receptionist should have alerted staff as soon as she saw Mae standing at the door with her stuff. What should be a facility's policy on this or similar situations?

3. What accountability policies are appropriate for residents in facilities, e.g., under what circumstances should caretakers keep track of residents?

4. Are caretakers given formal training about what procedures to follow when a person is missing? If so, what are they? If not, what should they be?

5. Many people in a community do not know others who live there. It may be because they have moved to a new retirement community or a care facility or because so many of their old friends have moved away or died. The elderly can feel like they're with strangers, or like they're outsiders. With that in mind, consider and discuss how beneficial it would be for a facility to:
   a. Ask a couple of established residents to intentionally look after for a new resident when he/she first comes.
   b. Have a staff person assigned to a new resident as a "buddy" that first week or month.
   c. Have *all* staff be part of a "buddy system" so that *each* resident within your facility has a staff person as a buddy. What would be the benefits to those staff who normally do not have direct resident contact? What would be your facility's expectations of staff in this role? How would you set it up?

6. In a way similar to question 5, how can a community act so the elderly still feel like they are an active part of what is happening?

Who Cares about Dancing Angels

1. At a community meeting, do some brainstorming and come up with a list of the most commonly asked questions that the elderly have in regards to their daily needs.
   a. Once you have your list, prioritize them in rank of importance (the first time, from a caretakers' perspective; the second time, from an elderly person's perspective.) Once you have the two lists, compare and discuss.
   b. Which of those items in 1a does your community have

a good track record of dealing with on a timely basis? Which need work on?

2. When the elderly person's care schedule, therapy, etc., conflict with a desire to attend other activities, how is that resolved? Is it different based on where the person is living?

3. Who is responsible for assessing an elderly person's weekly schedule to make sure the necessary things (meals, baths, etc.) are getting taken care of? How should conflicts with activities that person enjoys going to be resolved?

4. If an elderly person is in a situation where care conferences are held, do these care conferences routinely address the issues in questions 2 and 3? If no, would there be any benefits *for the caretakers* in doing so? Discuss.

5. Who deals with the spiritual issues of the elderly? (This can be a significant problem when people can no longer go to worship services outside of their home or when they are in a facility without a chaplain.) Have the people who are trying to provide these services received any training in this area? If not, how could that training be provided?

6. Discuss: How important would it be to have either a part-time or full-time minister to see to the spiritual needs of the elderly in your community.
    a. Does your community see spirituality as a vital component in providing care for the elderly? If so, how is that manifested?
    b. What benefits would a minister be to the caretakers themselves? In what ways would you use a minister?

The Sandwiched Generation

1. Are care conferences you participate in based primarily on the medical model (dealing mainly with medical issues such as changes in medication, therapy needs, etc.) or do they address the whole person? Explain.

   a. Do you ask the subject of the care conference and/or the family to fill out an evaluation form on the care conference once it is concluded? If so, who looks at it and decides how this information is used?

   b. Would such data (la) be valuable to you? In what ways? What kinds of questions would you like to see on it?

   c. Once the care conference is completed, what kind of follow up is given on concerns expressed by the elderly and their families?

   d. Who has the responsibility of annually reviewing *the process* of how care conferences are done?

   e. If you could change anything about the way care conferences are done, what would it be? How could you go about doing so?

2. What kinds of surveys (of families/elderly) are done in your community? Do you have access to the results of those that may be of some benefit to you? If not, how would you get such access? What kinds of surveys would you like to see done?

3. The expression "the sandwiched generation" was referred to in the story, and how those affected are so often stressed-out, emotionally exhausted, and physically drained.

   a. How many of the caretakers you know are in the sandwiched generation? What kind of support would be helpful to them? (e.g., providing day care for the children of the caretakers, having a caretaker "relaxation" area, etc.).

   b. What services (counseling, support group, training) are

provided for those caretakers (3a)? Discuss how this would be of benefit.

The Car's in the Garage

1. Make a list of things you have heard the elderly say that you consider to be symbolic language, e.g., "I want to go home." often refers to dying and going home to God. What kind of training is offered to caretakers to help them understand the symbolic language of residents, e.g., Daisy's "car in the garage"?

2. Do some brainstorming on how caretakers and families may unintentionally contribute to loss of independence for the elderly. Make a list.
    a. You may wish to use a group of the elderly as a focus group and ask them the same question.
    b. Once you have the list, discuss how changes can be made *and* how you increase caretaker awareness and sensitivity to this.

3. Review your community's policies and physical layout, looking at its effect on independence. What can you do to increase the independence of the elderly? How can this benefit others in the community, too?

Love has no law.

— *Portuguese Proverb*

Love Birds

"Love birds" was the expression a staff person used to describe the two of them. "That's what they are, just a pair of love birds." It was an apt description of Neal and his wife, Iris — and Neal considered it to be a joy living up to. He took delight in telling others, "Iris and I have been married sixty-eight years," adding with the fervor of one just married, "and we're still in love." When he was asked whether the two of them had ever had an argument in all those years, Neal just smiled and said, "Oh sure, but the secret for a successful marriage is to argue a lot and nobody wins."

Iris was admitted to our nursing home after Neal decided he could no longer care for her at home. Having had no children nor close relatives with whom to confer, Neal simply decided one day that it was time and called for an appointment to come in to make the arrangements. Looking back, Neal can tell you the day and exact time he made the decision, but he will also add that it was something he had known in his heart for months. He knew what he had to do, but he also said it was a traumatic and heart-wrenching experience to do that to his wife. This was especially the case since he recalled that when they were in their sixties, Iris had made the comment that she would never want to be in "one of those places." Neal had shared his wife's comment with the staff while doing the necessary paper work the morning Iris was admitted. He told them that his wife's statement had come after the two of them visited her second cousin in a nursing home. Iris had told him that her cousin didn't want to go to that place, and "had been tricked into doing so by family members who told her she was going to see the doctor." According to Neal's account, what made it even worse for Iris was that the nursing home was so run down and smelled so bad that a person got depressed just walking through the front door. That one experience made such a negative impression on Iris that after her cousin died, she never again wanted to set foot in any nursing home. In her opinion, they were nothing more than human warehouses for those who, abandoned by their families, had nowhere else to go. She also was convinced that the reason her cousin died so shortly after she entered the nursing home was that she could not stand to live there. At the time, Iris made Neal promise that he would never put her in a nursing home.

"This will the one and only promise I hadn't kept to her in all our years of marriage," Neal sadly told the staff when he was signing the necessary papers to have his wife admitted.

By the time Iris came to our facility, she was disoriented to the point of being completely unaware of her surroundings. As far as she was concerned, she was still in her bed at the senior citizen high-rise apartment where she and Neal had been living for the past fifteen years. Besides exhibiting the effects of dementia, Iris' physical condition had declined. She was so weak that she barely had the strength to sit up in her bed to eat. For the past two months at home, Neal had bathed, dressed, and fed his wife. He also had cleaned her up after her accidents. Changing the bed linen was difficult but Neal said he managed. In addition, he did the cooking, laundry, and other household chores. To keep from disturbing his wife at night, Neal slept in a lounge chair that he had paid some kids to move into the bedroom. At age ninety-four, Neal reluctantly admitted he could no longer keep up with everything and still give Iris the care she now needed.

Neal's doctor had strongly encouraged him to place his wife in a long-term care facility and even given him the telephone numbers of several he recommended.

The staff was deeply touched by the devotion Neal showed his wife. Though he lived nearly fifteen miles away, Neal drove in to see Iris every day. That mileage may not seem like a long distance, but we were all concerned about Neal's driving since he wasn't in the best of health himself. Besides, we knew that his doctor had suggested to him that perhaps it was time to give up driving. Neal considered it, but said he felt he could not as long as Iris was so far away from him. "I have no one to depend upon to drive me," he informed us. The only days Neal missed coming were those when weather advisories recommended no driving because of snow or bitterly cold temperatures. On those days, he called the nurses' station to check on how his wife was doing, reminding the staff to make sure Iris took her medication. A few times when he telephoned, Neal persuaded a staff person to go to Iris' room. He would then ring his wife's room, having instructed the staff person to answer the phone and hold the receiver to Iris' ear so that she could hear his voice and not be lonely.

I can only imagine what Neal must have said in those phone calls to his wife. Having observed the two of them together on several occasions, however, I speculate the call going something like this:

Hello dear. It's your husband.

No verbal response, but Iris opens her eyes.

I'm sorry, but I can't come in today. It snowed out last night, and the roads aren't plowed yet.

No response.

Do you remember the time in our first year of marriage when it snowed so much that we got snowed in for three days?

A hint of a smile crosses his wife's face.

I'll never forget that, dear.

Iris closes her eyes. She is also remembering.

I know you can't talk, but I wanted you to hear my voice. I told the nurses about your medication. You be sure to take it.

Her eyes open.

I love you, dear. Get some rest now. If it doesn't snow any more, I'll be up tomorrow and we'll talk some more. I miss you.

Iris's lips part as if she wants to speak, but no words come.

Bye, bye, dear.

As I was making my rounds one day, I came upon Rebecca, a housekeeper who had just come from Iris' room. As I said, "Good morning," I noticed that Rebecca had tears in her eyes.

"Rebecca, what's the matter?" I was afraid that perhaps Iris had died. Many of the staff knew that Iris' condition was poor. A couple of them had already made comments, saying how sad it would be when Iris died because Neal would be lost without her. Even though Rebecca and other staff are not in direct care giving to residents, they do find themselves deeply caring for the people they see on a daily basis as they clean their rooms, bring them their laundry, or replace the bulbs in their lamps.

"Oh, I just finished dusting the room," Rebecca replied as she put away some supplies in her cleaning cart. "Neal is holding Iris' hand, and talking to her. Her eyes were open, but she wasn't responding." Rebecca sighed. "That man is so devoted to his wife and has shown so much love." She took a tissue to dab at the tears that were now on her cheeks.

"I understand," I replied, trying to comfort her. "It's sad, but they've had a good life, and Neal told me he has many fond memories of their years together."

"It's not that," Rebecca said.

"What is it then?" I asked.

"It's just that," she paused and took a deep breath, "I'm not sure my husband would do the same for me."

Special Places – Special People

They can be verbally and even physically abused. They work at jobs that cause many people to wonder how they put up with the stress day after day. Physically, the work is demanding, and their bodies often suffer the consequences; very few last to make it a life-long career. Hardly a glamorous job, they are the ones called upon to clean up the messes when residents have accidents or get sick to their stomachs. In between cleaning up the messes, they are also constantly transferring residents from bed to wheelchair, from wheelchair to bed, from bed to toilet, from toilet to wheelchair, and so on throughout the day. Although countless hours are spent in training about proper lifting techniques, it is a job that inevitably takes its toll.

Who are these special individuals? At our facility they are called NARs (Nursing Assistant, Registered). At other facilities, they may be referred to simply as nursing assistants. Regardless of their title, they are the backbone of the long-term care industry.

They are the ones who feed, bathe, clothe, toilet, and groom; these tasks are done day after day, and often times, under trying circumstances. These individuals tell stories of being punched, slapped, or even choked by confused residents who didn't want these "strangers" around. One shouldn't think that the elderly are always weak and helpless. I remember an incident several years ago when it took two police officers and a male staff person to subdue a woman in her eighties who was physically attacking residents and staff. On another occasion, a staff member related how her fingers were nearly broken when a resident, suffering from hallucinations, grabbed her hand with such a powerful grip that it took two other staff to pry his fingers back to release her.

Once, after a meeting, I had the opportunity to talk with a group of NARs. We talked not only about how physically hard the work is, but also about their emotions when those for whom they care, die. They would want it to be known that although they are considered professional caregivers, they get as much from those for whom they care as they themselves try to give. When someone dies, it is often like losing a member of their own families. They will admit the work can be difficult and that they will never get financially rich from what they do; yet, they will also say with pride that there is a reward they receive that is far beyond what is brought home in their paychecks.

It just so happened that two in the group of NARs I had talked with had been, that very day, subjected to some racial slurs from two different residents. Unfortunately, these kinds of things happen on a regular basis. When asked about these latest incidents, Diane, one of the two, responded, "It's hard, but I try not to take it personally because I know it's their age. One minute they can call me a name but the next minute they have forgotten all about it."

"And you still take care of them?" I asked, wondering what I would do if I were in similar circumstances.

"Oh, yes," she replied and then, after pausing, added, "It hurts, but I do it because I love and really care about them even though they may not always know it."

Nate, the other NAR, also targeted by the racial slurs, shared some thoughts I know would represent the attitude of many of his peers. "I take care of them as if they were my own grandmother or grandfather," he said, speaking quietly. "I always try to treat them with respect."

I have often heard people say, "It's got to take a pretty special person to work in a nursing home."

Personally, I couldn't agree more.

Winning the Sweepstakes

Vilma told the nurse that she wanted to talk to the chaplain. "Tell him it's not urgent, but I think he'll be interested in what I'll have to say."

When the nurse relayed the message to me that same day, she commented, "By the look on Vilma's face, whatever it is she wants to tell you, it seems pretty important. And not only that," the nurse added, with an expression on her face as if she had just seen the eighth wonder of the world, "she was smiling! Can you believe that!" she exclaimed. "Vilma was actually smiling." The nurse paused and shook her head in amazement. "I don't know what's come over that woman in the past couple of weeks, but let's just hope it stays."

In the two years Vilma has been a resident at the Home, the staff members have never seen her smile. One housekeeper said that she thought she had noticed the hint of a smile one day after she had complimented Vilma on the colorful dress she was wearing. Whether it was the beginnings of a smile, though, the housekeeper could not be sure. "Maybe it was only heartburn," she had joked.

To say that Vilma has had less than a warm and cheerful personality would be an understatement of significant proportions. In the past, she had turned aside any efforts from the staff to get her involved in activities with other residents. "I prefer to keep to myself," she replied every time an invitation was extended to attend a resident activity. The only time she was with others in a group was at meal times when she sat at a table with two other residents. There had been a third person, but he decided to sit at another table after only two weeks. He told his new tablemates that it was like sitting under a dark cloud with Vilma at the table. The two residents who presently sit at the table with Vilma are individuals who also keep to themselves, although they are seen at some resident functions.

I went to visit Vilma the day after the nurse gave me her message. As I knocked at her door I was wondering what could have taken place in her life to cause the apparent change that the nurse had noticed. I was also curious about what she had to tell me and what connection it had, if any, with the frequent smiles staff and residents were now noticing about her. Vilma had once told me that she often sends in her name for the various sweepstakes contests she receives in the mail. Whereas other residents enter and joke about receiving a check for a million dollars, Vilma is quite serious about winning and feels that it is only a matter of time. It is no wonder that she is sitting and waiting every morning by the resident mailboxes for the mailman to show up. When he does show up, she is there, asking if there are any "official looking" envelopes for her.

Vilma answered my knock at her door, and while there wasn't any hint of a smile on her face, there was definitely something different about her; the frown and doleful expression she usually wore were gone, and the lines in her face seemed softer. It could have been my imagination, but there was even an air of graciousness surrounding her. In addition, she looked a good ten years younger than her true age of eighty-six. There was no question in my mind that this woman had gone through some kind of transformation, and I remembered asking myself at the time, if winning ten million dollars could do that to a person and deciding, beyond a doubt, it could.

"Good day, Chaplain," she said in a tone of voice that was inviting and friendly. "Won't you have a seat?"

"Good morning." I walked over to the chair she had shown me and sat down. "You're looking good," I said as she took a seat across from me.

"Thank you," she cheerfully replied. "It's nice of you to have come. I would offer you some tea and a cookie, but I'm afraid I'm out of tea bags and haven't had the time to do any baking this morning."

It was only until Vilma smiled that I realized her comment about not having the time to bake was an attempt on her part at humor. "That's okay," I said, "I'll take a rain check on the cookies." I was amazed at the change I was seeing in this woman.

"I have something to share," Vilma announced, "and I thought of all people, you as the Chaplain, would like to hear it."

"I surely would," I replied, thinking that maybe she did win some money.

"Good," Vilma said. "I was reading an article in the paper a couple of weeks ago; it was in the Sunday edition. It was a story about the ill effects of holding on to grudges and past hurts. It was written by a woman who hadn't talked to her daughter for over seven years." She paused for a moment. "The daughter had done something when she was in her early twenties that terribly hurt her mother's feelings. Her mother felt it was unforgivable and would not speak to her daughter." She stopped, eyed me, and then asked, "You didn't, by chance, see the article, did you, Chaplain?"

"No, I guess I missed it."

"The daughter was killed in an automobile accident," Vilma continued. "At first, the mother wasn't going to go to the funeral but changed her mind when other family members talked to her. When the mother saw her daughter in the casket, she broke down completely, realizing how much she had missed in their relationship for those seven years. The article was written by the mother. It was a very moving piece and it hit me like a bolt of lightning from the sky." She paused for a moment. "After reading it, I decided it was time to write a cousin of mine."

As Vilma continued her story, she talked about how she and her cousin had gotten into a terrible argument years ago. They both had said things to one another that were very vicious. Whatever had been said to Vilma, she had been deeply hurt and had had no dealings with the cousin for nearly nine years. According to Vilma, each had felt she had been wronged by the other and was waiting for the other to make the first move. However, after reading the story, Vilma decided that she needed to do something since she didn't know how much time she had left. "At my age, death could come at any time," she said.

"I wrote a letter to my cousin three weeks ago," Vilma shared. "In it, I apologized for anything I may have said or done to hurt her. I also asked her to forgive me." She took a deep breath before going on. "I didn't know how she would react to what I had written, or if she would even write back. All I knew is that after reading the article, I had to write. And when I mailed the letter I felt such a sense of relief. It's just something I can't explain." She took another deep breath and smiled; there was a look of peace upon her face.

"That's some story," I said.

"But, wait, Chaplain, there's more. Guess what I got in the mail three days ago?" Without waiting for any answer, Vilma reached over to the nightstand next to her chair and picked up an envelope that was lying by her telephone. "This is from my cousin. She thanked me for my letter and said she needed to rethink the past as well. She didn't come right out and apologize for anything, but she did say she would call me next week." Still holding the letter, Vilma smiled again.

Everyone has noticed the change in Vilma. She, for her own reasons, however, has not told others about the article or the letter she wrote to her cousin. Many of the residents and staff wondered what had come over her. A few even wondered if she had won the sweepstakes. I think, perhaps, in a way she has. What do you think?

Gone Fishing

"When I die, I'm going fishing," Bernard announced to me as I sat with him and his friend Everett at their table. It was during their breakfast time, and the three of us were having coffee.

"I'm going fishing, too," Everett piped up, not to be outdone.

"You can't," Bernard replied gruffly as he helped himself to a second spoonful of sugar and stirred it into his coffee.

"Why not?" Everett shot back just as gruffly.

Bernard took a sip of his coffee, swirled it around in his mouth as if he were tasting fine wine, and then placed the cup back on its saucer. He scratched his chin, picked up his spoon, wiped it with his napkin, and then dipped the spoon into the sugar bowl. Only after he had stirred in his third helping of sugar did he answer his friend. "Because, Everett," Barnard growled, giving his friend a stern look, "I've already explained that to you and you know I'm right! Just ask the Chaplain, here. He'll tell you."

Little did I know that that Tuesday morning when I decided to visit residents in the dining room of the Board and Care section of the nursing home that I would find myself in a discussion about death and fishing before I finished my first cup of coffee. When I stopped at the table where Bernard and Everett were sitting, I was invited by both of them to pull up a chair and have some coffee. The conversation certainly began innocently enough: the weather, how to fix the squeaky wheels of Everett's walker, the new resident on second floor who looked too young for being eighty-five. After the two of them agreed that the new resident must have been lying about his age, the subject of fishing came up. That, too, began innocently enough.

"Chaplain, did you go fishing this summer?" Bernard asked.

"I'm afraid I didn't," I replied as I sipped my coffee. "I'll just have to wait and go next year."

"No fresh fish; that's too bad," Bernard replied. He took a bite of his toast and chewed it thoughtfully. "You know something, Chaplain; nothing's as good as fresh-caught fish."

I nodded in agreement as I took another sip of coffee. Everett, I noticed, had put his cup down, and looked as if he wanted to say something.

Bernard spoke up again, "But Chaplain, did you know that I once ate fish that were nearly three years old, and they tasted as good as if they had just been caught that same day."

"Really," I exclaimed, wondering if he was about to tell me some "fish" story. "How was that?"

Bernard poured some coffee into his half-filled cup and picked up his spoon. This time he did not wipe the spoon as he dipped it into the sugar. Only after satisfying himself that his coffee was sufficiently sweet enough for drinking did he reply. "Easy," he said. "Put the fillets in a milk carton, fill it with water, and then freeze it. They'll keep forever, and the fish will taste fresh." He wagged his finger at me, "You have to try it sometime, and you'll see for yourself."

It was at this point that Everett cleared his throat loudly and spoke up, telling me that he and Bernard were having this disagreement about how Bernard had tried to tell him that he couldn't go fishing after he died.

I looked at Barnard, "How is it that you can go fishing when you die and Everett can't?" I hoped that this wasn't some kind of judgmental statement Bernard was making, as if he were implying that where Everett was going when he dies, there is no water. Although Bernard and Everett were the best of friends, Bernard could be very opinionated about religion and matters of faith.

"That's easy, Chaplain," Bernard answered, wiping off his spoon again. "That's because my grave has a pond near by, and so, I'm going fishing."

"And what about Everett?" I asked.

"Like I told him, Chaplain," Bernard said. "He's on the other side of the cemetery. There are no ponds around him, not even close. As I explained to him, you can't go fishing where there's no place to fish." He glanced over at Everett before looking back at me. "Isn't that right, Chaplain?"

"But I want to go fishing," Everett pleaded. "And I don't see why I can't."

At this point, I wasn't sure if this was a serious discussion or if they were just *baiting* the chaplain to have a little fun. Yet, Everett did look upset. I thought to myself that either Everett really is upset or he is the world's best ninety-three-old actor. Thankfully, I didn't have to solve the dilemma. Whether it was my presence or merely the number of spoonfuls of sugar Bernard had put in his coffee, Bernard softened his position as he said to his friend, "Everett, I tell you what. When that time comes for both of us, I'll come by and pick you up whenever I go fishing. Okay?"

"That sounds good to me," Everett said.

"Thank you, Chaplain," Bernard said. "I knew you'd help."

"Yes, thanks," Everett echoed his friend.

"Anytime," I replied as I got up to leave, figuring this was as good of a time as any to depart before any other discussions came up.

"See you, Chaplain," Everett said.

"Bye, Chaplain," Bernard smiled and then added, "Don't forget about putting the fish in milk cartons."

"I won't." As I walked away, I heard Bernard say to Everett, "Pass the sugar, will you; don't be hogging it."

Questions for Reflection

These questions are meant to be catalysts, to stimulate creative thinking about ways at providing quality, holistic care for the elderly. In some instances, the reflecting may lead to new (perhaps untraditional) ways of providing care. Not all questions may apply to your situation, but *all* situations will benefit from reflecting upon them. Whether your community is a long-term care facility, a new retirement home, or the old neighborhood, you can adapt them to fit your situation.

Love Birds

1. How does your community recognize/celebrate wedding anniversaries? What additional ways could it be done?

2. Discuss celebrating wedding anniversaries of people whose spouses *no longer* are living. What could be beneficial for the

living spouse in doing this? What are appropriate ways to do this? Consider, e.g., having (with the person's permission) a picture display of their married life together — houses they lived in, trips they took, children, grandchildren, etc. Discuss how this might benefit caretakers, too.

3. Neal talks about a certain nursing home he visited that was so bad that he got depressed just walking through the front door. If you are part of a facility that cares for the elderly, you might want to consider the following:

   a. What kind of first impressions is given to those who visit your facility?

   b. Consider inviting a group of people from the surrounding neighborhood to tour your facility. After they are finished, use them as a focus group and ask them the following questions:

      1. What did you like about what you saw, heard, and smelled?

      2. What did you dislike about what you saw, heard, and smelled?

      3. Would you put your loved one in our facility? Why or why not?

   c. Do a walk through your facility and list the unpleasant smells and sights you see? Discuss whether your furnishings, lighting, decorations, etc. make you feel happy or depressed? What could be done to improve your facility?

   d. Have members of the staff (throughout the whole facility) anonymously fill out a questionnaire asking the same questions from 3b, 1-3.

   e. Based on the feedback from questions 3b and 3d, how would you rate your facility?

   f. If actions need to be taken to improve your facility's environment, whose job would it be? Will they have the necessary power and authority to make the changes? Discuss what the following means: The empowerment of staff.

g. Since everyone always talks about the "bottom line" (what will it cost?), considering questions 3a to 3f, discuss the following: The best marketing plan for our facility is the facility itself. Consider also: Are staff part of the marketing for a facility? Discuss.

4. Being with Iris every day was very important to Neal. How can your community help couples stay together when health concerns require them to live in different places much of the time?

Special Places – Special People

1. The story is based on the assumption that nursing assistants are vital to the long-term care industry and the care of the elderly in other situations, too. Therefore:

    a. In what ways is the importance of their work formally recognized within your community (e.g., having a "Nursing Assistant Week")?

    b. Do a focus group with nursing assistants and ask them to list frustrations of their work. Once they have the list, ask them to prioritize it.

    c. Discuss concrete ways the top five frustrations in 1b can be reduced.

2. Diane and Nate talked about prejudices. Do you feel there is prejudice within your community? Explain. If there is, what steps could be taken to reduce it?

    a. What kind of training are caretakers given to deal with prejudices of the people they care for?

    b. Have the prejudices within your community been addressed (both between caregivers and the people they care for *and* between different caregivers)? If they have not been addressed, why not? Whose job is it to do so?

    c. If a certain person continually makes racial slurs toward caregivers or other members of the community, how do you handle that? Are there written policies on it?

    d. Discuss the benefits of having a nursing assistant support group where they can get together and talk about the stresses they experience with their work.

3. One of the nursing assistants talked about taking care of residents as if they were his own grandmother or grandfather. Discuss how that philosophy may be encouraged for other caregivers?

4. In many parts of the country caregivers have a different first language than the people they care for. This can often lead to complaints by the elderly that they can't understand what the caregiver is saying because the accent is hard to understand. Does this need to be resolved so that the elderly know what their caregivers are saying? How can this be done?

Winning the Sweepstakes

1. Vilma changed her attitude toward a certain relative after reading a newspaper article about the ill effects of holding on to grudges and past hurts. Assuming family dynamics affects your elderly and caregivers:

    a. What kind of training do caregivers feel would be helpful to them as they deal with the elderly and their families?

    b. How is the family member who is consistently verbally abusive to caregivers handled?

    c. Discuss the inherent problems of caregivers avoiding certain difficult people and/or family members.

2. How would your caregivers handle the following situations:

    a. A person tells you that he had an argument with his son and doesn't want anything more to do with him. The person tells you not to call his son under any circumstances. That night, the resident has a heart attack and is near death. The only person listed as family is the son. Do you call?

b. The family places, in your opinion, unrealistic expectations on their father who requires a significant amount of care. As a caregiver, you see the father become depressed after each time the family visits. Do you talk to the family? Should anyone talk to the family? If yes, who?

c. Two elderly people have an argument in an eating-place. One of them slaps and pulls the hair of the other. Fortunately, neither one is seriously injured, but this is not the first time they've fought. How should the situation be handled? Does it make a difference whether the people involved are in a long-term care facility dining room or are fighting in a downtown restaurant? Why?

Gone Fishing

1. In this story, the chaplain took time to have coffee with two residents. Discuss the benefits of caregivers sitting down and talking with the elderly from time to time outside of normal care situations. What might the caregivers gain? What might the elderly gain?

2. Bernard and Everett talked about going fishing after they died.
    a. In what ways do you intentionally have opportunities for the elderly to talk about end of life issues?
    b. If you do not have a chaplain or minister available, who might facilitate such a discussion group?

3. What kind of end of life issues do you feel the elderly you know deal with?

4. Would it be helpful for caregivers you know to have some basic training in dealing with the issues you listed in question 3? Explain.

Who gives to me, teaches me to give.

— *Dutch Proverb*

A Command Performance

Every week Sam (he prefers to be called Sam rather than Samuel) provides special music by playing the piano for the worship service in one of the wings of our Alzheimer's Care Center. Sam himself is one of the residents in the Center. By his own admission, he isn't a particularly religious person. Yet, by his own choice, he is there every week for the service. He learned the piano as a young man, and regularly played in piano lounges wherever he lived. It wasn't his full-time job but his avocation. Sam loves to play the piano. It is part of who he is.

"Do you think God will like what I play?" Sam asks as he slowly rises from his chair to take his place at the piano. For Sam, it is not a frivolous question.

"Of course, Sam," I reply. "God will enjoy it."

Sam smiles and looks pleased that he is about to play for such a prestigious audience as God. Knowing Sam, he will perform as if he were performing before a packed concert hall; or perhaps a more suitable analogy, he will play as if he were playing in a crowded piano lounge with standing room only. As Sam reaches the piano he pauses, looks at me, and asks, "Are you sure?" As he asks his question, he points upward, surmising I would know whom he was asking about.

"Yes, Sam, I'm sure."

Sam adjusts the piano seat and sits. He stands up again to move the seat ever so slightly, and after he sits again, he lightly fingers the piano keys without producing a sound. After stretching his arms, he announces he is ready. It is a ritual he no doubt acquired over the years. There is no need to adjust any sheet music as part of his ritual since Sam plays from memory. I nod to give him the go ahead, and before I get a chance to sit down, Sam is already pounding out the tune *Alley Cat*. It is one of three tunes he usually plays for God, often times mixing the melodies of all three. Those in attendance, however, do not notice nor seem to care because they are too busy tapping their feet. I can imagine God doing likewise as Sam glances up toward the ceiling every now and then.

We have a sixty-bed Alzheimer's Care Center at our facility. It is divided into three wings or pods as they are sometimes called. Each wing has an all-purpose room referred to as the Great Room. On this morning we are using that room for our worship. Once the service is over, the residents will stay for coffee and cookies served by volunteers. This afternoon the residents will gather in that space for one of their favorite activities — bingo. At other times during the day, the room is used for exercises, watching television, listening to music, reading the paper, or doing jigsaw puzzles. Besides these activities, the room also serves as an area for the residents to pace in and out of throughout the day and, as can be the case of those with Alzheimer's, throughout the night as well.

The wing where, this morning, we are hearing *Alley Cat* is the South Wing, the wing where Sam is a resident. Those who live there are in the middle stages of Alzheimer's. Those who reside in the North Wing are in the advanced stages while those in the West Wing are in its early stages. While those with Alzheimer's can prove to be difficult to handle in any given situation, Sam's friendly smile and engaging personality always has a calming effect upon those who have come for the worship service. He is seen as a nice person who loves to give of himself to others by playing the piano; it is part of who Sam is.

Sam became a resident several years ago after his family reluctantly decided that they could no longer take care of him. Although Sam had physical problems due to the natural process of aging, that was not the determining factor for placement. It was his increasing symptoms of dementia that made the decision necessary. Sam's continual pacing at all hours of the day and night, along with his irregular sleep habits, were draining family members of their energy. What little energy they had left was quickly used up when he began to wander outside without regard to weather or his own safety. That proved to be the last straw. As one of his family members said, sighing in a voice too tired to care whether she was heard, "The emotional and physical energy … I just ... just didn't have any left to worry about his safety."

Placing Sam in the Alzheimer's Care Center was an agonizing decision for the family. It was made only slightly easier because Sam's adjustment to his new home went relatively smoothly and because he was now in a secured environment. With his various aches and pains, Sam realized that, as he said with a laugh at the time of his admission, "I'm not as young as I used to be." Family members noted that it was his way of expressing that he realized that something was changing in his life.

If you were to visit with Sam, you would find him to be a personable man who likes to talk about the traveling he has done in his life. Over the years, Sam traveled all over the world with his work, and continued to travel in his retirement years. Proud of his trips, he has several photo albums of the places he has been. If you expressed even a hint of interest, Sam would get the photograph albums from his dresser drawer to share the pictures of the countries he had visited.

Although he only occasionally remembers where the photographs were taken, he does recognize himself in them, commenting that the picture was taken when he was younger. As for the other people in the photos, including his family, he shakes his head and confesses with a half smile, "I don't know who they are. I guess I don't remember so good anymore." Sam sometimes continues to stare at a particular photograph before turning the page as he tries to remember who those *strangers* are that were standing next to him.

When Sam sits down at the piano to provide the special music for our worship service, I never know what he will play, nor do I always recognize immediately what he does play because of his tendency to blend the tunes. Besides *Alley Cat*, he usually plays *Mexicali Rose,* or *Let Me Call You Sweetheart*, and upon occasion, other mixtures of tunes that neither I nor the music therapist recognize. After he finishes playing, we show our appreciation by applauding. Sam bows, looks upward with raised bushy eyebrows, and with his hand above his head, he points toward the ceiling and bows again.

"Do you think God liked that?" he asked me after he had taken his bows and was shuffling back to his chair to sit with the other residents.

"I know God enjoyed that," I replied.

"That's good," Sam replied, smiling. "I enjoy playing for God."

When Sam plays *Alley Cat*, we use it as a lead-in to talk about cats, dogs, canaries, and any other pets the residents may have had when they were younger. The message I try to get across is that all of these creatures are part of creation, and thus, are reminders of the Creator. We do the same with *Mexicali Rose*, only we talk about the many varieties of flowers within creation, and, as a follow-up, we sing the old-time favorite gospel hymn *In the Garden*. The tune *Let Me Call You Sweetheart* presented a little more of a challenge, but it was decided that this is simply another way of God expressing love for us. All of these connections might raise a few eyebrows among professors and students of theology, but they are meaningful connections and bring smiles of acknowledgment from those in the South Wing of the Alzheimer's Care Center, especially to a piano player by the name of Sam who feels privileged in being the opening act for God. Playing the piano for God is part of who Sam is now.

4000 Hours and 3 Gallons of Blood

She is not a resident, but those who live at our nursing home love Helene and accept her as part of their family. Her story is worth being told because within it there is a clue that will help you answer the question: How can I find meaning and purpose in life? Helene has found the answer for herself, and she will tell you what works for her can also work for you.

At age seventy, the joints in Helene's fingers are beginning to have the familiar ache associated with arthritis, and although she has a hearing problem, she'll tell you it's not so bad that she needs a hearing aid — yet. While there are those who still entertain the stereotype of a person Helene's age as someone spending her time in a rocking chair and knitting, they might be surprised to learn that Helene doesn't own a rocking chair, nor does she have any immediate plans for buying one. And any knitting she does is done on the run. Helene doesn't have time to slow down because she is too busy fulfilling one of the most important roles at the nursing home and within her life — being a volunteer.

Individuals like Helene enable nursing homes across the country to provide a quality of care that would not be possible were it not for volunteers. Helene, for example, comes nearly every day, volunteering between twenty and twenty-five hours a week. Her dedication is evident as she was recently honored for having reached 4,000 hours of volunteer work. Among the many things she does as a volunteer are bringing residents their mid-morning coffee and cookies, reading the newspaper to them, pushing their wheelchairs, writing their letters, reading their mail to them, giving them hugs, and laughing and crying with them. With all the things she does in her role of volunteer, one could easily understand how the residents love and need her. Helene, however, would say that helping the residents provides meaning and a sense of purpose for her life, too. She says without hesitation, "I need them just as much as they may need me."

While having coffee with Helene one day, we talked about why she volunteers. Her responses provide some insight into her as a person, the kind of values she has, and where those values came from.

"I'm a widow and there's nobody home," she says as she sips her coffee. "I just enjoy being with the residents and talking with them."

"So, you get a lot of pleasure visiting and being with them?" I ask, already suspecting how she'll answer.

"Oh, yes!" Helene exclaims. "I love to listen to them talk because they have such interesting backgrounds, and they have done such marvelous things. You can't look at them as old people sitting in wheelchairs." As she speaks, there comes across a note of deep respect for those whom she is talking about. "They have climbed mountains and swum oceans," she points out. "They're fun to be with. With all the physical things going on in their lives, they still have such a wonderful sense of humor. I get more from them than I think they get from me."

"What happens when they die?" I asked, knowing how close Helene becomes with the people she cares for. "Isn't it hard?"

She took another sip of her coffee and reflected for a moment. When she speaks, it is with quiet reverence. "When someone dies, I think of it as a part of life. The minute we're born, you know, we're moving toward death. It's not easy," she says sadly. "Of course, I don't want them to continue suffering, but it's hard." She paused, wiped away tears, and then explained, "Right now, I'm thinking of friends who have died. I'll never get used to it. I don't think a person should ever get used to it."

Helene went on to talk about how she began volunteering as a young married woman. After her husband died, she turned to volunteering almost full time.

"You have always done volunteering, haven't you?" I said.

She nods her head and smiles. "It's another way of caring for others. I learned the value of giving from my parents who came to this country around the turn of the century. They were so thankful for their new country that they decided they would give something back." As she speaks, I can hear the pride that comes from serving in her voice. "Both mother and father volunteered thousands of hours to various organizations and causes over the years."

"So that's where the seed was planted."

"That's right," Helene acknowledged, "and I think they instilled this value within me for a purpose."

"And that would be?"

"I think they knew it was important for me to know that volunteering gives a person some meaning and purpose in life."

Toward the end of my conversation with Helene, I asked, "Have you ever thought about the time when you may become a resident?" Her answer reflected her inner beauty and wisdom.

"Oh, yes. I've talked to my children about that. My daughter wants me to come live with her, but I told her it would be better if I went into a nursing home." Helene smiled and then offered this statement that, for her, is a call to others to find the answer to the purpose of life as she has. "I hope that there'll be a volunteer who will do the things for me that I try to do for others."

If you think Helene's philosophy of helping others is only confined to the residents of a nursing home, you need to reconsider. The morning I had coffee with her, she was wearing a tee shirt given to her by the Red Cross. The shirt read: Thanks for having given three gallons!

A Vision in the Night

Deathbed conversions occasionally come up during discussions about faith and spirituality. When they do, they usually make for interesting conversation. Although such conversions are supposed to be quite common, I personally have never been present at one. Even now in my role as a chaplain where I have sat at the bedside of many dying people, I have yet to be a witness to a conversion. What I have witnessed, though, is that those who know that they soon will be dying can and do have spiritual experiences right up to the very end. Such was the case of Frieda.

Frieda had been a resident in the Chronic Care Center for nearly three years before she died. Although she liked social contact, she didn't have much interaction with other residents because many of them have hearing problems, and Frieda was so softspoken that her normal tone of voice was barely above a whisper. She had a number of medical problems that are too numerous to go into, and as Frieda once remarked, "They would only bore a person," adding, "Who would want to listen to an old lady talk about failing kidneys and how she hates wearing a diaper?" On another occasion, she summed up how she was doing by simply announcing, "I'm fighting life." Though Frieda's body continued to fail her, her mind did not. She was constantly asking questions concerning spiritual matters. Her questions didn't come because she was doubting the existence of a power greater than herself, but rather she wanted to keep herself on the growing edge of what she felt was her inner spirituality. One of her favorite expressions was "You never stop growing," and then she would add with a laugh, "even though my body's shrinking, I'm still growing."

"I had a vision the other night," Frieda told me one afternoon as we visited in a lounge area. I had sought her out after a nurse had mentioned that she had earlier asked to see the chaplain. "You know, I've had visions all my life," Frieda continued, as she settled back in her wheelchair, shifting what little weight she had.

"I know you have," I replied. In previous visits, she had shared how her spirituality had, at times, manifested itself in visions. It was a part of her spirituality that was important to her, and she often mentioned it.

"This vision had something to do about a house in heaven. The house was beautiful and so peaceful." Frieda closed her eyes for a moment as if she were revisiting the vision. "Do you think God is trying to tell me something?"

"Could be," I said. "I don't know. What do you think?"

"I'm not entirely sure," Frieda said. "It sure was peaceful. I figured it might have something to do with my body telling me that it will soon be time to go."

I took notice that her face looked gaunter than it did the last time we visited just a week ago. "Are you worried about that?" I asked.

"Of course not," she quickly but calmly answered. "What do I have to be worried about?" Frieda shifted her weight again. "This old body is worn out. I'm ready to go but I'm just waiting on God's timetable." She looked at me with a questioning eye. "He's sure taking his good old time about it, but that's okay since he's given me this new vision. I've something to ponder until that time comes." Frieda paused and then, looking me straight in the eyes, said assuredly, "I know where I'm going."

"When you get to heaven," I said with a smile, "save me a place."

"You do your own saving," she replied with a laugh.

I was anxious to learn more about her spirituality. "Where do you think these visions and the questions you have come from?"

"What else have I got to do?" Frieda asked. "I'm not physically able to do the things I used to," she stated unemotionally. "I can't see to read or to watch television. Besides," she groaned, "who wants to watch that stuff on television, anyway. It's just mindless junk." She wrinkled up her nose and patted the arm of her wheelchair. "The visions and thoughts just come to me as I sit in this thing. This darn old chair will outlast me." Frieda stopped for a moment, and then suggested, "Tell you what, Chaplain. You can have it after I'm done with it."

Frieda was a person who spoke so softly that I had to be within twelve inches of her, and even then, it was difficult to pick up all the words she was saying. When I asked about her soft voice, she smiled and said that she inherited it from her mother who had a voice that was, "softer than cotton candy."

"I get down, you know," Frieda said, her eyes peering at me through her wired-framed glasses.

"Over what?"

"Oh, how people treat each other. There's so much unfairness in the world." Before going on, she stopped to watch two nursing aides who were helping a resident walk. The male resident was groaning with each step he took.

In our conversation, Frieda shared that she had been an observer of people all of her life. I noted it was something she continued to do as she observed the daily interaction between residents and staff, residents and residents, and between staff. She frequently pointed out how certain staff members approached their work. For example, she told of a male aide who did his work, but who really didn't care for the people he was helping. She said that he wasn't comfortable being around "us old people." Asked how she knew that, she simply replied, "I just know." Frieda also cared about the other residents, and she told me that day we talked how another resident was very depressed because of a recent stroke that left her unable to speak. Frieda said she was worried about her and wished she could do something for her.

"Sometimes I get so confused about life," Frieda said as the two staff people helping the resident to walk turned the corner of the hallway. We both could hear the groaning sounds coming from the resident who was having difficulty walking. "I have questions but don't seem to get any answers. I sometimes wonder why God allows such things as pain and getting old."

"I wish I had the answer to that but I don't," I replied.

"You know, Chaplain, most of us who live here don't mind getting old, but we don't like getting old and being *sick* all the time." Frieda shifted her body in her wheelchair; she, I knew, was in constant pain herself. She was so frail and thin that her bones looked as if they could break through her skin at any moment. "What I really wonder about is why people treat each other the way they do." She shook her head as if to emphasize her statement. "I think God is telling me something with that vision I had, but I'm not sure what it could be. I'm still pondering it."

I knew that Frieda, given enough time, would unlock the key to her vision. "Let me know what you come up with, okay?"

"Sure," Frieda replied. She grew quiet for a moment. "You know I've had religious experiences all my life."

"Really?"

"Yup," Frieda replied. "I had one when I was ten years old." She didn't elaborate but said, "Maybe it was gas." She chuckled at her comment, and then added in a serious tone, "But I don't think so."

Knowing Frieda, I don't think so, either. This woman of spiritual visions died, and I never did find out what she came up with after pondering her vision of that peaceful house in Heaven. I do know, however, that her spirituality never ceased to provide her with new growth experiences right up to the day she died.

A (Darn Good) Storyteller

"They're trying to poison me," Lester would exclaim as we sat in his room with the door shut. So convinced that *they* were out to get him, he would have locked the door if it was possible. During the whole time we visited, he kept a watchful eye on the door, every now and then, explaining, "Gotta be careful. You don't know who may be listening to us out there."

If you had ever had the opportunity of meeting Lester, you would have understood how he might easily have qualified for anyone's list of the *Ten Most Unforgettable Characters I Have Ever Met.* From his storytelling, to his taste in clothing styles, to his views on certain kinds of foods, and to his paranoia about gravy and aluminum cookware, Lester was unmatched. Any one idiosyncrasy would have given Lester the label of *character,* but when all of these were combined, the result produced an individual who is not easily forgotten.

To have a memorable experience, one only needed to spend some time with Lester as he spun one of his yarns. It soon became clear how Lester might well have been the role model for the expression: "He could talk your arm off." Lester would not only talk your arm off, but your leg as well. The only problem was that he had such a pronounced drawl that even if you would have pleadingly offered your leg on a platter, he would never quite get to it. He thought of himself as a *darn good* storyteller and he was, in his own unequaled way. The uniqueness of his storytelling came mostly from the manner in which Lester told his stories. He would interject long pauses between phrases to emphasize a point he was making. As if the pauses were not enough, Lester would often grin like the Cheshire cat in Lewis Carroll's *Alice in Wonderland.* He grinned whenever he felt he had made or was about to make an important point, and for him, that was about every third phrase. The trouble with Lester's storytelling was that he never got around to finishing his tales. He certainly had no problem in getting the listener's interest, but just as it was piqued he would start going off on one of his tangents. He would begin to describe minute details to the extent that he seldom got back to the original story. One day, for example, he began telling me a story about a relative who had served as a drummer boy during the Civil War. He was at the part in the story where this young lad set out from some place in the Midwest on a march to Washington, DC. The story started as a very interesting tale, but as usual, Lester got off his subject. He began by describing how blacksmiths in those days had to forge steel into bands that strengthened and helped keep the wagon wheels together. After twenty minutes of listening to a detailed description of the forging process, I said that I had some other residents to visit. "I had planned to stay for only a short time," I pleaded. As I got up to leave, Lester took hold of the sleeve of my suit coat and firmly tugged; it was his way of informing me to stay put.

"Now, I'm not finished telling this story ... (long pause) ... I'm just coming to the good part ... (big grin, long pause) ... you just sit down in that chair," he said, still holding on to my jacket sleeve, "and we'll get on with the story ... (big grin)."

After another fifteen minutes of wagon wheel construction, I took advantage of a pause to get up, this time making sure I was beyond his reach. "Lester," I shouted (he was very hard of hearing), "I'm sorry, but I really have to leave."

Lester looked at me and raised his pencil thin eyebrows. "Why, I was just coming to the part on how the wheels were mounted onto the wagons ... that's mighty interesting ... (grin, long pause) ... I guess I'll have to tell you tomorrow ... you're going to visit me again, aren't you? An old man like me needs a visit ... (big grin) ... I've got a darn good story to tell you. A darn good story."

"I'll come back, but I don't think I can come tomorrow," I shouted as I inched my way toward the door.

"Well, I'll see you tomorrow ... yes, sir, that march to Washington, DC is mighty interesting ... (grin, long pause) ... mighty interesting ... guess you just have to come back to hear the end of the story ... (big grin). You'll be surprised at how it ends."

Along with Lester's unique style of storytelling, he also had his own unique style of dress. His entire wardrobe consisted of plaid sport jackets and pants, and whatever he selected to wear was always a mismatch. As much as staff tried to help him coordinate his clothes, he turned aside their suggestions, telling them, "Nothing wrong with these clothes ... had them for a long time ... I think they look pretty sharp ... I could tell you a story about them, if you want … you might learn a bit about fabric …" Lester's clashing plaids were so much a part of him that staff could not honestly remember him in any other style of clothes in the fifteen years he was a resident.

Another side of Lester that certainly would contribute to his being a memorable character was his ideas about food and how it was to be cooked. He refused, for example, to eat anything that was cooked in an aluminum pot. When I asked him why, his explanation was in detail about the history of aluminum, and according to him, the studies done on how it affected food cooked in it. He cited magazines and journals that I've never heard of. His explanation was so long that very few staff, myself included, could hear it out to the conclusion. One of the housekeepers was determined to hear Lester's full explanation, and one day decided to hear him out. After forty-five minutes, however, she had to leave to resume her duties. When asked about it, she sheepishly admitted she had lost track of what he was talking about in the first ten minutes.

My first encounter with Lester's theories about food came about when I asked him if he liked gravy on his potatoes. That, as I learned quickly, was a big mistake. As staff later told me, Lester had been a long-time staunch opponent of gravy because he "knew" it to be poison. Again, no one could figure out exactly what he had against it, but woe to any new staff person who would serve him meat or potatoes with gravy. On more than one occasion, he asked me to come to his room to discuss a matter of great urgency. I knew the routine. As I came in, he would say, "Shut the door. I don't want anyone to hear."

"What is it Lester?"

"They're trying to poison me again," he would claim, and then go into an explanation of how he was served gravy with his meat at dinner. "They're out to get me," he would whisper.

Olive oil also played an important role in Lester's culinary peculiarities. The nurses' station was always stocked with an ample supply of olive oil that Lester had personally purchased. He would ask for a bottle every few days, take it back to his room, shut the door, and drink it. The reason? "It cleanses the plumbing system," he explained with a smile.

I believe there is one other reason why Lester could be considered unforgettable, and that is for the *gift* he left behind. The legacy he left was a piece of scrap paper on which he had written a question. It had been given to one of the nurses many years ago and was brought to my attention by another staff person who somehow had acquired it and who had posted it on the bulletin board in her office. She showed it to me a few days after Lester had died. Lester's question, "Do you ever visit the old and sick?" was a reminder to her of the reason she got into this kind of work in the first place.

Since Lester had no family, and had outlived all his close friends, the staff had their own Service of Remembrance for him a week after he died. The informal service was held in a conference room on the floor on which he had been a resident. The room was filled with staff that had come to share memories and reflect upon what this man had meant to them. There were tears, of course, but more laughter as we remembered his storytelling, the mismatched plaid jackets and pants, and his ideas on cooking in aluminum pots. A moment of reflective silence occurred, however, when the scrap of paper upon which Lester had written his question was passed around. As the staff read it, one could sense that what he had written was a reminder to all who were there of their common humanity.

Can't you almost feel Lester's tugging at you and saying as you were handed that scrap of paper with his question written upon it. *Sit down awhile. This is something to ponder. You might learn something ... there's a darn good story here ... (long pause, big grin.)*

Save a Dance for Me

Balloons and other decorations were everywhere. A twelve-piece band was playing one of Glenn Miller's tunes from the

1940s, *A String of Pearls*. Nearly all the two hundred plus people in attendance were wearing some kind of party hat, and the noise-makers that had been passed out as people arrived were already being put to use before their appointed time. The big affair was the annual New Year's Eve dance at the Home, and all were enjoying themselves. Among those celebrating was Laurette. She was on the crowded dance floor being twirled around by her dance partner. The look of delight upon her face was matched by those who were watching Laurette relishing the occasion. Her warm glow showed how much she was enjoying the dancing, and for a few magical moments, she was able to lay aside the many problems that the aging process had presented her.

Laurette has been a resident for nearly five years, living most of those years in the Chronic Care Center. She had initially resided in Board and Care, a more independent section, but it was only a few months until a stroke had left her partially paralyzed. Her stroke required a move to a unit that provided the staff care she now needed. Much to her dismay, her speech had been severely affected and her mobility greatly limited. Through intensive therapy, however, she regained enough of her speech so that if the listener works hard at listening, Laurette could be understood. According to the speech therapists, further improvements for her would be only minimal. Not being able to express herself as she had in the past is very frustrating for her. She becomes very anxious about expressing her thoughts, and consequently becomes unable to string together even two or three words, let alone a complete sentence. At the peak of her frustration, all she can manage to say is, "Help. Help. Help."

The effects of Laurette's stroke have naturally been very depressing for her, and she readily admits being "down in the dumps." It's embarrassing for her to be involved in social events with other residents because very few of them can understand what she is saying. While many of the other residents are sympathetic, they are not always careful about hiding their own frustrations with this woman they are trying to understand. Laurette therefore chooses to spend time by herself. It took a great deal of encouragement and time for staff to persuade her to attend the New Year's Eve dance.

The dance is held in the mid-afternoon, and residents from all parts of the facility are invited. The music is provided by a band that plays the tunes of the 1940s. According to many of the residents who are in attendance, the tunes of the 1940s are the only kind of music that is suitable for dancing. Besides staff, there are a number of volunteers whose primary purposes are to be dance partners for any residents who wish to dance. Much to the delight of the residents, and adding to the ambiance of the event, the female volunteers dress up in evening gowns and formal party dresses while the male volunteers are in tuxedos and black ties. After the dance, light refreshments are served. For the residents, it is a celebration that brings back memories. The party concludes with the singing of a song that unites all who are in attendance — *Auld Lang Syne.*

Laurette was sitting at a table with others, but she wasn't attempting to be part of the conversation. She looked very much alone. When I first approached and asked her to dance, she looked at me for a moment as if I had to be out of my mind. She shook her head saying, "No ... no ... I don't ... uh ... think ... uh ... uh ... so." Having declined the offer, she turned and looked toward the band.

I noticed Laurette's foot tapping in time with the music. Remembering having been told by the music therapist that Laurette had been sometimes persuaded to attend the sing-a-longs that were held on the unit where she lived, I decided to take a different approach. I wasn't sure where it would go, but I just didn't wish to walk away. "Laurette, do you like the music?" I asked.

As soon as I asked the question, Laurette turned her head so that her eyes met mine, "Oh ... uh ... yes ... yes." The look on her face gave me the impression that my question was unnecessary, as if to say, who wouldn't like this music. There was some change in her eyes, perhaps a spark that encouraged me to try one more time in asking her to dance.

"Why don't we give it a try and get out there for one dance," I offered with a smile. "If you don't like it, or if you get tired, I'll bring you back. Okay?"

Her eyes fixed on mine for a long time. I wondered what was going on in her mind. What was she thinking? I hoped that she wasn't considering going back to her room. Perhaps, she was regretting even coming. Maybe she was hoping I would just go away and leave her alone. Was I embarrassing her? Putting her in an awkward position? Maybe this was a stupid idea on my part in the first place. Before I could speculate any further, I saw another change in her expression, a liveliness in her eyes as she replied shyly, "O ... O ... uh ... kay."

As Laurette and I went out onto the dance floor, I was aware that others were watching us. The staff from Laurette's floor had been especially concerned about getting her more involved socially with others. They no doubt were pulling for her, hoping that the New Year Eve's gathering would give her some self-confidence in groups. They knew, as I did, that the aftereffects of a stroke — paralysis and speech impairment — make a person quite self-conscious.

Laurette and I managed to have three dances in a row. During that time, she shared how she used to dance as a young woman. She loved to dance, especially at the dress-up affairs. I imagined her gliding around a huge ballroom floor with such gracefulness that all heads were turned toward her as she carried on animated conversations with her dance partner. When we got back to her table, those who were seated all complimented Laurette on her dancing. What was pleasing to see was how their smiles were met by hers.

To say it was extra special to dance with Laurette that afternoon would be an understatement, for you see, as I glided her around in her *wheelchair,* her eyes sparkled with joy and laughter. Perhaps, she was thinking back to another time, another place.

Questions for Reflection

These questions are meant to be catalysts, to stimulate creative thinking about ways at providing quality, holistic care for the elderly. In some instances, the reflecting may lead to new (perhaps untraditional) ways of providing care. Not all questions may apply to your situation, but *all* situations will benefit from reflecting upon them. Whether your community is a long-term care facility, a new retirement home, or the old neighborhood, you can adapt them to fit your situation.

A Command Performance

1. Sam's family talked about how hard it was to place him in a facility:
   a. What kind of support is offered in your community to families with an elderly person who may need to go into a facility? Are there things that could be done that are not being done now?
   b. What support do the facilities in your area offer? What else could they do? If you are part of a facility, discuss what your plans are to meet the needs of resident families.
   c. Whose "job" is it to offer support to families? What kind of training could be given so that *all* of the people in contact with the elderly and their families are able to give support?

2. Sam had a photo album to share. Discuss benefits of having families putting one together for their loved one. How might the caregivers also benefit from this?

3. Discuss what your community could offer in terms of ongoing educational opportunities for families dealing with Alzheimer's?

a. Who offers such educational opportunities to your community?
b. What would be the benefits of offering such programs as 3 and 3a? Who would be responsible for starting such programs?

4. If you do *not* have a music therapist available, in what ways are you using music to help the elderly? What could be done that isn't being done now?

5. What other kind of sensory experiences are you providing for your elderly? e.g., smells, touch, and hearing (familiar sounds such as trains bring back memories).

6. Evaluate living quarters for Alzheimer's: Would you put your loved one there? Why or why not? What would you suggest to improve it? (If you're not sure, ask the families who have relatives in an Alzheimer's unit).

7. Discuss the pros and cons of the following question: Should Alzheimer's residents be housed according to what stage of the disease they are in?

4000 Hours and 3 Gallons of Blood

1. Helene is a volunteer. Her work, along with countless other volunteers, is invaluable to the lifeblood of any facility. Volunteers also are vital in community programs for the elderly.
a. How do you *now* recruit volunteers for a program you are involved in? Whose job is it? Is it a priority?
b. Brainstorm *innovative* ways to recruit volunteers (e.g., placing ads in the newspaper, or offering incentives to those who recruit volunteers).

2. How are volunteers presently given recognition within your organization?

    a.   Who is responsible for doing so?

    b.   What are the needs of your volunteers? Who formally accesses their needs?

3. Helene talked about how she was affected when a resident dies. How do you help volunteers deal with death when someone they have closely worked with dies?

4. When Helene was asked about what she saw in her future, she said she planned to move into a nursing home rather than move in with her daughter. There are other possibilities, such as in home care. What do you think the best solution is? How does it depend on the physical and mental state of the person needing care?

5. What presently unmet needs of the elderly could volunteers meet? What activities and opportunities could you make available or expand if you had volunteers?

6. Have *each* department in your facility or each community service program you are part of answer the following questions:

    a.   How could *we* benefit if we had all the volunteers we wanted? (If you haven't historically made use of volunteers, challenge yourselves as to how you might use volunteers.)

    b.   Do we simply ask for volunteers to help out with existing programs or do we visualize new programs that could be done and then recruit volunteers to help us fulfill that vision? Discuss at length.

    c.   What kind of visionary programs do we have for the future that people will volunteer for because they are excited about them?

A Vision in the Night

1. There are residents (like Frieda) whose minds are sharp and who need to be challenged.
    a. What kind of programs/activities do you have now that challenge/stimulate residents intellectually and spiritually?
    b. What could you be doing?
    c. What would the elderly you know like to see that you presently are not doing?

2. Frieda could tell that a certain aide really didn't care for the people he was helping. Discuss the following:
    a. If, as a caregiver, you knew of another caregiver who was doing his or her job mechanically (without caring), what would you do?
    b. In the face of stress and burnout, how would you help caregivers maintain compassion over the years?
    c. Some will argue that compassion cannot be taught, but the question for you is how can it be intentionally *nurtured* among the caregivers you know?

A (Darn Good) Storyteller

1. Lester's question "Do you ever visit the old and sick?" was a reminder to a nurse why she got into the work she does. Have caregivers discuss why they got into the work they do. (We have many seminars on the how-to's of our work but few on the why's.)

2. The story talked about a Service of Remembrance where staff (as well as family members and other residents) had the opportunity to share memories and reflect upon what Lester meant to them.
    a. In what ways would such a Service of Remembrance be valuable for caregivers involved with the person who

died?

    b. How are caregivers you know given an opportunity to have closure for those who have died?

3. If you decided that a Service of Remembrance would be helpful, who could facilitate it? Where would it be held?

4. Residents like Lester demand a lot of time from staff in the telling of their stories:
    a. Discuss the benefits of having some basic training in setting time boundaries. (Without basic training, caregivers could come across as being rude or uncaring.)
    b. As far as setting time boundaries, how might that be helpful with meetings? What could be done to have more effective/productive meetings?
    c. Discuss the benefit of learning time-management skills?

Save a Dance for Me

1. Laurette suffered from low self-esteem because of her stroke. In what ways can staff help promote resident self-esteem? Discuss the benefits of having resident support groups. Who could facilitate such a group? What would be the purpose?

Character is a line on stone; none can rub it out.

— *African Proverb*

Scrapbooks

Even if you never have had the opportunity, have you ever wondered what it would be like to visit "the old folks" in a nursing home? If you ever had the opportunity, would you have some apprehension about making such a visit? Are you concerned that you would have trouble finding a topic to talk about with residents who are in their eighties or nineties? Do you think that the only things the elderly would want to talk about are their aches and pains?

If you answered *yes* to any of the above questions, then I have just the person for you to visit. His name is Martin. The reason I suggest him is that, first of all, you would enjoy visiting with him. Secondly, you wouldn't have to wonder whether you would have anything to talk about since Martin would have plenty of things to share. And thirdly, you wouldn't have to worry about his complaining about his aches and pains — he won't, although he has his share of them. He would be gracious enough, however, to listen to *you* complain about yours; that is, if you don't go on and on.

In his late eighties, Martin would delight you with stories of the many fascinating things he has done over the years, charm you with his subtle sense of humor, and intrigue you with his philosophy of life. If you visit with him, though, plan to spend a couple of hours because Martin will share with you what he considers to be his most prized possessions — his scrapbooks. The hours spent looking through his scrapbooks would be some of the most enjoyable time you would ever spend. For Martin, it would also be enjoyable because he would get a chance to talk about his life in its entirety and, therefore, be seen as more than just an "elderly" person. For yourself, it would be enjoyable because you would pleasantly discover how many of those who reside in nursing homes are so ageless. In addition, it may surprise you just how much you have in common with people like Martin when it comes to life's hopes, dreams, and values.

Martin came to the Home two years ago after deciding that he was beginning to slow down. He talked about how his eyesight was failing and how he reluctantly gave up driving. Approaching his eighties, and walking with a cane because of increasing unsteadiness also had something to do with his giving up his apartment and moving into our facility. "Us older folks got to make room in the world for the younger ones coming up," he quipped. His wife had died five years earlier, and although his two sons each invited him to live with them, Martin declined, explaining, "They have their own lives to live."

The first time I met Martin was in the Town Square, an area of the Home where residents can gather in a variety of settings: a coffee shop, a library that has several reading tables, and a game room where there are card tables and a billiard table. Martin was in the coffee shop having a hot fudge sundae. After introducing myself, he and I talked for a few minutes about how he was adjusting to his new surroundings. He told me he loved being at the Home and then asked if I would stop by his room when I had the chance. He had something he wanted me to see. "Chaplain, I think you might enjoy looking at it."

A couple of days later, I knocked on his door. I found myself quite curious as to what he was going to show me.

"I'm glad you came," Martin said, showing me a friendly smile. He invited me in and told me to get the chair from his desk and sit next to where he was sitting.

We hadn't talked more than five minutes when Martin got to the reason he had wanted me to come. "I want to show you something, Chaplain," he exclaimed as he pointed to the right of me. "It's over there by the bookstand." I looked but I wasn't sure what I was looking for. "It should be on the bottom shelf," Martin said. "It's a green album. Do you see it?"

"Yeah, I do," I replied as I got up and went over to the bookstand. Printed on the album's cover are the words, "My Scrapbook." The 11 x 14 album is two inches thick and heavy enough that I needed both hands to lift it. As I did, I took note of another scrapbook underneath it. By now, Martin had moved my chair closer to his. I sat down and laid the book on my lap.

"Open it up." Martin sounded like someone who had just given a present and was waiting with excited anticipation to see the person's reaction as he unwrapped it.

I opened the album to the first page. There was a certificate scotch-taped to it; the tape was yellowed with age. The certificate, though a bit faded and had what appeared to be watermarks, was still legible. As I examined it closer, I saw that it was a certificate for perfect attendance in Sunday school. It was dated 1913.

"This is a pretty old document," I announced as I glanced up at Martin. "And you've kept it all these years."

"Yes sir, and I'm pretty proud of it. I was the only one that received a certificate that year. Of course," Martin added with a small chuckle, "there were only thirteen kids in the whole class." He pointed to the certificate. "Did you see the signature? It was signed by the Sunday School Superintendent."

Martin went on to tell me stories of the church he attended for most of his youth, how religious his parents were, and the one (and only) time he sat in the front pew of the church on a Sunday morning.

"First time I ever did that was when I was about eight or nine years old. I watched the minister climb up into that pulpit. That man looked like he was ten feet tall. He was a nice man, I guess, but he preached Hell and Damnation. He was what we called in those days, a *pulpit pounder*."

"Did he scare you?" I asked, trying to imagine Martin as a little boy.

"Scare me?" Martin said, chuckling. "Why he scared the ... ah, he scared the tar out of me that day. That old preacher looked right at me when he talked about the fires of Hell." He chuckled again as he slapped his knee. "I never did sit in that front pew again."

In the next forty-five minutes or so, Martin and I got through no more than five or six pages of the scrapbook because of the stories he told that accompanied the certificates, letters, cards, photographs, and news clippings. Through his scrapbook, I was getting to know Martin. The book documented all the things that he considered to be important. Each page was a testimony to the fullness of his life. Each item the scrapbook held served to broaden my view of him rather than seeing him as just a white-haired old gentleman with failing eyesight, walking with a cane.

Just as I enjoyed my visits with Martin, so would you. Once you had completed all your visits with him, looked through his scrapbooks, and heard his stories, there are other residents I would like you to meet. They also have their own *scrapbooks* to share. Blanche, for example, has a spoon collection that she and her husband collected in their travels, beginning with their honeymoon and ending with the last trip they took before her husband died. After Blanche, then you can visit with Milton. He has a collection of model tractors that are reminders of his life on the farm. He spends hours sharing stories, some dating back to the mid-1800s when his parents homesteaded in the Dakotas. He will tell you about horses and plows, about life in a sod house, and about how grasshoppers nearly wiped them out one year. Next comes Erma. You can visit with her and see her collection of oil paintings. The paintings, which she did herself, have an unusual theme; they all are of outhouses. Imagine the stories Erma could tell. If you have time, then you need to visit with Elsie. Her room has a beautiful mahogany china cabinet against one wall. Its beauty is surpassed only by the charming collection of teacups. "Each cup has a story," Elsie points out when you visit her and take notice of the collection.

The next time you visit someone in a nursing home, whether it's your first time visiting with a certain individual, or whether you have visited before, keep a discerning eye open for the scrapbooks, whatever form they may take. There are delightful and interesting stories behind them. If you see no scrapbooks, then ask about their *verbal scrapbooks*. Ask them about what Christmas or Thanksgiving was like as a kid, or the first car they rode in and what that was like.

Ask about their first experience with indoor plumbing, their first job, the smells they remember from their mother's kitchen, or their first day in school, or…

Are you still wondering what it would be like to visit "those old folks" in a nursing home? Do you still think there wouldn't be much to talk about? Do you still wonder if all the elderly have to talk about is their aches and pains?

If you still need convincing, there is one other person I would have you visit. It is Sherman. His "scrapbook" is a collection of empty cereal boxes.

Uniquely Unique

A week before she died, Bessie was still curiously intrigued with why so many people thought of her as being a *unique* personality. "What makes me so unique?" she would ask the staff. As far as Bessie was concerned, in all of her eighty-six years, she had thought of herself as being quite ordinary.

That Bessie was anything but ordinary was shown by how she handled hearing the results of a biopsy taken from a lump discovered during her routine checkup. Her doctor informed her that she had a fast-growing cancer. Furthermore, the doctor explained that because the cancer had metastasized, surgery was not an option. The aggressive chemotherapy suggested was declined by Bessie after she was told that the treatment had only a ten-percent success ratio for this type of cancer. Besides the low success rate that treatment offered, her decision was also influenced when she learned of the potential side effects of it. Always a neat and proper lady, the thought of hair loss was not appealing to Bessie. She said she would never look good wearing some type of turban, and a wig would only make her head itch. If the pain could be controlled, Bessie explained to the doctor, that would be sufficient; all she desired was to die with some dignity.

As Bessie related to me, before she left the doctor's office that morning, she thoroughly quizzed him as to what she could expect in the time ahead. She asked him what vital organs initially would be affected, the kind of pain medications he would prescribe and why, (Bessie, to the doctor's surprise, was quite knowledgeable about pain medications) and lastly, what would be the probable cause of death since she understood that cancer, per se, would not be listed as the reason on the death certificate. After being informed that death would most likely occur because of kidney failure, Bessie, in her dry wit, replied that she was not surprised since she had always had weak kidneys. Throughout the doctor's explanations, Bessie listened with the same interest and intensity she had when she had attended lectures at college in her younger days. Her questions were intelligent and her comments, knowledgeable. All her life Bessie had been interested in the pursuit of knowledge, and she saw no reason to change now. Although I have no verification, I wouldn't be surprised to learn that when Bessie left the doctor's office that day, she left him thinking to himself: *Here I prepared myself to break the news to this woman that she is dying, expecting to make use of my bedside manner to comfort someone who I thought would be overcome by shock. Instead, I end up feeling as though I just gave a lesson to someone who shares my fascination with the field of medicine. What an interesting, unique individual.*

Growing up during a time when opportunities for women were limited, Bessie's uniqueness surfaced as she was determined to better herself in every way. She devoted her energies to becoming "a career girl." Marriage was never an option because, as Bessie confessed, she never really took the time to know any man well enough to consider it. "Besides," she said without a hint of self-pity, "my looks were a drawback." Tall and gangly, Bessie never considered herself an attractive woman. "I know that I'm not a good-looker," Bessie said in her characteristic candor, and then added, "I also seem to intimidate men. You know, of course, I'm reasonably intelligent and I speak my mind. I've found that men do not always like that from a woman." In exhibiting her intelligence and speaking her mind, Bessie soon discovered how easy it was for men to be threatened. She became disenchanted with the business world and found a fulfilling career working in the field of education as an executive secretary to a college president. The work atmosphere and college setting were both intellectually stimulating and sufficiently challenging.

Although Bessie never would consider herself a gifted person, her talents were many: she spoke German, French, and enough Latin to get by; she loved classical music and could name the composer and piece of music within the beginning moments of hearing the piece; she taught herself to play the piano, but not well enough to meet her own high standards. Along with these gifts, Bessie also was accomplished in oil painting and sketching. She did both landscape scenes and portraits, preferring, the latter. One afternoon while we were visiting in her room, I asked if I could see some of her work. She instructed me to open the bottom drawer of her dresser and take out the large manila folder underneath several other smaller ones. Once I removed all the folders, she gave me very specific instructions in placing the other smaller folders back into the drawer. It was obvious that Bessie had her own way about things. She was meticulous about having a certain order within her life. Enclosed within the folder, each individually wrapped in protective tissue as well as carefully separated by layers of tissue, were a dozen of her drawings. Unwrapping them, I made a mental note how the tissues were folded so that I could refold them in exactly the same way. As for her sketches, I only needed to look at the first few to appreciate her talent. After I had seen all of them, Bessie asked me if I wished to look at some others that were under her bed. She explained that they were too large to store in the dresser drawer. Before getting them out, however, she wanted me to put the ones I had just looked at back into the manila folder. I was in the middle of rewrapping the first one in its protective tissue when Bessie spoke up.

"Chaplain, I'm afraid that's not right," she pointed out, gesturing toward what I was wrapping.

"What do you mean?"

"The way you're wrapping it," she explained. "The left side of the tissue is folded first, and then the right side goes on top of it." She paused and gave me a slight smile. "You have folded the right side in first."

"Oh, I see," I replied, although I really didn't understand what difference it made. I followed her instructions and was just placing it back into the folder when Bessie again spoke.

"Chaplain?"

"Yes, Bessie."

"I see you're about to put the drawing in the folder with the top down. That's not correct," she said, gently wagging her finger at me. "The bottom of the drawing should be put in first so the bottom is at the crease of the folder. It was that way when you removed it."

"Thank you, I'll do that." Now I had a hunch that this was going to be a long process; and, unfortunately, my hunch turned out to be right. For the next fifteen minutes I was given step-by-step instructions how each drawing, once it was properly wrapped, was to be replaced into the folder. My assumption that each drawing would be inserted the same way as the first, of course, proved to be mistaken. When it came time to put the folder back, I had quit making assumptions and simply waited for Bessie's directions. I knew there would be another set of instructions for returning this folder to its proper place among the others. I was right; there was. By the time we had finished, if Bessie had asked me again how I thought she was unique, I would easily have had a reply.

Bessie died within three months of being told of the biopsy results. A group of staff and residents gathered to remember her one afternoon. It was an opportunity not only for all of us to have closure, but also to share stories and reflect upon this woman who had so touched our lives. Each person who attended had a story about Bessie and how she was one-of-a-kind. Perhaps, though, Yvonne, a trained medication aide, shared the one story that best revealed Bessie's uniqueness. She related the following conversation she had had with Bessie two weeks before Bessie died. It took place one afternoon when she had stopped to give Bessie her pain medication.

"Yvonne," Bessie began with a warm tone, "I just want you to know you've always been special to me."

"You're special to me also," Yvonne replied.

"What's so special about me?"

"You're just a very unique person, Bessie."

"That's what the chaplain said. That I'm unique." Bessie got a puzzled look on her face. "What do you mean by *unique?*"

"You've always been interested in the world, its events, and our lives. I have appreciated how you always ask about my family. You're also very intelligent, and you have your very own sense of style."

"But I was always such a tall, gangly thing."

"If you were born now-a-days, you would have been a fashion model."

Yvonne said that Bessie thought about that for a moment and then replied with a sense of humor and her typical candor, "I might have made it as a fashion model, but I would definitely have needed breast implants."

Upon hearing that story we all agreed that only Bessie could have come up with a line like that.

My Friend Flicka

"Hey, Poik, where are you going?"

I didn't have to turn around to know who was calling me; it could have been none other than Flicka, one of the most delightful residents I've ever had the opportunity to meet. Her given name is Zelma but after the first time our paths crossed, I would call her Flicka, and she would call me Poik. When I initially inquired what poik meant, she winked and then replied with a mischievous look on her face that reflected, I soon was to discover, her fun-loving spirit. "Oh, that's Swedish," she told me. "Poik in Swedish means *boy*. So, that means you're a poik." Her bright smile and sparkling eyes were infectious and I felt myself taken in by her charm.

In her early eighties, Zelma had moved into the Home just two days prior to our initial encounter on a warm and humid Monday afternoon in July. Our paths crossed in the hallway. She had just come from her room. For most people moving into a long-term care facility, there is often a difficult period of adjustment in the first couple of weeks. Some people take months to adjust; others never adjust; and then there are those exceptions, like Zelma, who settle in from the very first day. Zelma was determined to make the best of things, and did so with enthusiasm for her new home. She had a zest for life that those much younger would envy. When Zelma, for example, began using a walker a few years later, she continued to be such an energetic person that the staff amusedly wondered if they might have to install speed bumps in the hallways to slow her down. Zelma's enthusiasm for having a good time and making the most out of life was evident as she quipped when she first got her walker, "Do I need a license for this thing?"

"So I'm a Poik and that means boy," I had replied that first time Zelma and I met in the hallway outside her room. One of the nurses had told me about Zelma's fun-loving personality, saying that the new resident on second floor was a bundle of energy, and that I'd really enjoy her. I certainly agreed with the nurse's assessment as I asked Zelma, "What is Swedish for girl?"

"It's flicka," she replied, sensing that here was an opportunity to advance the cause of her beloved Swedish language. "You've heard that word before, haven't you?" she asked, giving me the definite impression that she was eager to make sure I knew.

"Flicka. Hmmm. Wasn't there a movie about a horse with that name?"

"You got that right, Poik. The name of the movie was *My Friend Flicka,* and you know what? It's about a girl horse." Zelma paused to let that piece of information sink in and then winked at me again before going on. "You know, you're a good kid. I think I'm going to like you," she said as she laughed. "You must be Swedish." Before I could respond, she walked away, and for a moment, I thought she was going to twirl her cane in a Charlie Chaplain imitation.

That initial meeting with Zelma took place several years ago, and although she is now slowing down, she is still as carefree as she was then. In spite of her declining physical condition, she remains positive about life, and the sparkle in her eyes has not grown dim. Displaying her usual great sense of humor, she is able to joke about the things happening to her. The other day, for example, she poked her head into my office and asked if I was busy. Without waiting for me to respond, she walked in and announced, "Poik, I'm not doing so good."

"What's the problem?" Wanting to hear more, I invited her to sit down. She wouldn't have come in unless it was something serious. I also knew that she would tend to downplay whatever was wrong. Zelma, like many residents, doesn't want to dwell on her problems by talking about them all the time. She was a person, though, who understands it is important to be able to share her problems with someone when she felt the need.

"Poik, I've got this inner ear problem," she said as she came in and stood in front of my desk, leaning on her walker. "It's been going on for a couple of months now. I don't know what is making me more dizzy — the medicine or the inner ear. I can't walk too good." I asked her to sit down again, and this time, she did. "My head feels as if it's spinning around," she told me. "I sometimes feel as if I'm going to tip over, like a ship tipping over on its side." She pointed to her walker. "That's why I have this thing now. I don't like it, but nothing I can do about it. I guess it's what happens when you get old."

"I'm sorry, Flicka."

"Oh, that's okay. I know you can't do anything about it, but I just had to tell you. I guess I'm just a dizzy blond now," she said and then added with a grin, "Except I'm not so blond anymore, am I, Poik? Thanks for listening." After she got up, she stopped at the door, flashed a warm smile, and said, "Poik, you're a good kid."

Trying to keep a positive attitude within the circumstances and not losing her sense of humor is characteristic not only of Zelma but also of many of the other residents as well. It's not that they are in denial of what is happening within their lives, but rather it is that they are trying to keep everything in perspective; the humor and laughter helps to provide a balance. It is a good balance to have since they live in a community where, on a daily basis, they see and hear the sights and sounds of people in poor health. They watch friends and neighbors succumb to the effects of dementia while wondering if that will also be their fate. With over 100 deaths a year within our facility, the residents know the reality of how fragile life is. They have had the experience of sitting at a table in the dining room when another resident had a stroke; they know what it's like to be awakened in the middle of the night by the movement of staff as they attend to the person in the bed next to them; they have seen the ambulances periodically come and go; they have also been witness to the funeral hearse driving away. Their use of humor and laughter is therapeutic as it helps them cope with such circumstances day in and day out. We all talk about living in a world of stress, but let us not think that those who reside in nursing homes are stress free. We could learn a few things about dealing with the stresses of life from our elderly. They could teach us, for example, about using humor and laughter to counter-balance those times of difficulty and pain, and they certainly could teach us the value of having a positive outlook. As one resident expressed it, "You can't always control the things that happen to you in life, but you can control how you react to them. Even though I'm in this wheelchair, I refuse to become a bitter old lady."

One of the most important things staff and visitors can do for those who live in nursing homes is also one of the easiest things to do as well — and that is to smile. Residents frequently comment how much they appreciate it when they see staff and visitors walking around with a smile. It helps the residents, and for two reasons you may not have realized: First, it shows them that the person is comfortable being in that kind of setting and truly enjoys being with those who live there; they are not simply seeing those with walkers and sitting in wheelchairs as "those poor, pitiful people." The second reason is that the smiles show the residents that they, the staff and visitors, have also discovered one of the ways to keep a balance in life.

A person like Zelma provides such a good role model. She is representative of the enduring quality of the human spirit and how it can survive even in the most trying of circumstances.

It has been said that when you feel sorry for yourself, you

should visit a nursing home. Unfortunately, the implication behind such a statement is that once you see all those poor souls, your own troubles won't seem so great, and consequently, by default, you'll feel better. I would suggest a more positive reason: visit a nursing home to learn from those who live there some ways in which one can keep a balance amidst the strains and stresses of life; to feel better because you discover from others that there are ways to cope with life, no matter what it may bring. A visit to a nursing home need not result in feelings of hopelessness, for there are many residents who are living examples of hope.

If you would like to meet an example of hope, there is this wonderful woman named Zelma — wait, you'd better call her Flicka. When you meet her, be prepared; she'll certainly charm you as she teaches you a few things about the benefits of smiling. She'll tell you in words, and show you by example, that life is to be lived to its fullest each day. Your visit with her will be made even more delightful if you should happen to know a word or two of Swedish.

The Leprechaun

"Hello in there," Einar hollered from the hallway. He was sitting in his wheelchair and peering in at me. Though the door to my office is always propped open to provide easy accessibility for people in wheelchairs or using walkers, Einar never enters my office whenever he stops to see me.

"Hello, yourself," I yelled back as I looked up from the report I was working on. As I got up to go out and visit with him, I had an inkling that Einar was up to something, and I knew I couldn't miss the opportunity to see what it was. He often had something to say that was *memorable.* "Just a minute, Einar I'm coming out."

"Glory be," Einar shouted, "it's about time you woke up from your nap." He chuckled along with the volunteer who was with him. I wasn't sure if their amusement was because of his comment or because of the two visitors who walked by at that moment and who were curious enough to steal inquiring glances into my office. As Einar sat there and grinned, I suspected he was up to his normal mischief.

As I later found out, the volunteer pushing Einar in his wheelchair had been specifically instructed to stop at the chaplain's office. "It's very important," Einar had told him. The two had come from the Chronic Care Center where Einar is a resident. They were on their way to the coffee shop that is located just down the hallway from my office. Coming to my office required only a slight detour. The impish expression upon Einar's face (he looked like a leprechaun who had just hid the pot of gold) told me that even if my office had been at the opposite end of the building, he would have had the volunteer make a *wee bit* of a detour to see the chaplain.

"I appreciate your stopping," I said to Einar, shaking his outstretched hand, and saying hello to the volunteer who had a bemused look. "To what do I owe this visit?"

"It's always nice seeing you, Chaplain," Einar said and then paused for quite some time. With his mischievous grin, twinkling eyes, and bushy white eyebrows teasing me, I could not help but wonder what was coming next. I was just about to say something when he asked me a question. "You know why I like seeing you, Chaplain?"

"No," I replied, trying to keep a straight face, "but I bet you'll tell me."

"That's what I like about the chaplain," Einar said to the volunteer who was obviously enjoying the playfulness of this leprechaun in a wheelchair. "Oh yes, the chaplain is always direct and to the point. Aren't you, Chaplain?"

"I try to be." I knew Einar was milking the moment for everything he could get from it, and to be truthful, he was good at it.

"Well, Chaplain, it's like this," Einar replied as his eyebrows twitched. "I like seeing you because that way I know I'm not dead yet."

When I laughed out loud, Einar just grinned and gave me a wink. Before I had a chance to respond, he motioned to the volunteer. "Let's go." Einar glanced back at me and waved. He was still grinning. No, it was more like a smirk — the kind that says: you can chase me, but you won't catch me.

Einar has lived at the nursing home for nearly three years. When he first became a resident, he was on the third floor of the Chronic Care Center. What precipitated his coming was that he had had a series of small strokes that caused some paralysis but did not affect his speech. After two months of therapy he improved to the point where he was able to move down to the second floor where residents are more independent. When told of the move, Einar remarked, "Well, what do you know? I graduated." The third-floor staff had been so charmed by this fellow that they had a going-away party for him. Einar loved it and was, to no one's surprise, the life of the party. " 'Tis nice that you throw this party for me," he announced. "You wouldn't have a shot of Irish whiskey, now?"

The first time I met Einar was on his second day at the Home. He came wheeling up to the nurses' station where I was writing a note to myself. The first thing I noticed about him was how his bushy eyebrows danced when he talked.

"Hello, my name is Einar," he announced in a brogue that was unmistakably Irish. "And who might you be?"

I introduced myself. As soon as he heard I was the chaplain, he grinned. There was something about the way he grinned that gave me an inkling that this person had a colorful personality and would prove to be a character.

"It's good to see a man of the cloth around here," Einar said. "Chaplain, I want you to know I love all people. It doesn't matter to me their race or religion. I feel love is very important."

"Well, I'm glad to hear that and..." I was about to compliment him on his attitude when he spoke up.

"Of course, the best kind of people are dogs and children," Einar said. "And Chaplain, do you know why they are the best kind of people?"

"No."

"Let me tell you." He glanced around as if he wanted to make sure no one was around to hear. "It's because of their innocence," he explained. "They're innocent creatures of the Good Lord. And they give you love back unconditionally." He nodded his head in agreement with himself. "I tell you, Chaplain, if more people were like children and dogs, we would have a better world. Big people are just idiots."

I wasn't sure how to take him. I didn't know if he was kidding or serious. "But, Einar, what about yourself, then? Aren't you one of the big people?"

Einar's eyebrows furrowed, and I wasn't sure what to expect. Suddenly, his eyebrows rose nearly to the middle of his forehead, and he grinned. "Chaplain, I have to admit you've got me in a corner." He paused as he stroked his chin. "Maybe some big people are okay," he admitted. Without saying another word, he winked and wheeled away with a quickness that surprised me.

Since our initial encounter, Einar and I have had many visits. I found out that he's a self-educated man. He quit school in eighth grade when his father died and went to work to help support his mother and a younger brother and sister. Although he never had any additional formal education, through life experiences and hard work, he, as he said himself, "didn't do so bad." Indeed, he didn't, since the last job he held was writing a column for a newspaper. When asked about what he wrote, he smiled and replied, "Old people like me." As I learned later, he wrote a column about concerns of senior citizens. Recently, he showed me an old newspaper clipping. It was an article about him upon his retirement in his mid seventies "to pursue other interests." The article praised him for his wisdom and stated that while he often "stirred the pot," he was always an advocate for the rights of the elderly.

Einar continues to make the detour to my office door. Just the other day I was working at my desk and heard his Irish brogue, "Anybody home?" Besides telling me again the reason he was glad to see me, he told me that he was thinking about suggesting that there should be a beauty contest for the "old ladies here at the Home."

"I don't know about that," I said, thinking that such a contest could prove troublesome in many ways. "Who would dare be the judge?"

Einar grinned, gave me a wink, and went on his way.

Question for Reflection

These questions are meant to be catalysts, to stimulate creative thinking about ways at providing quality, holistic care for the elderly. In some instances, the reflecting may lead to new (perhaps untraditional) ways of providing care. Not all questions may apply to your situation, but *all* situations will benefit from reflecting upon them. Whether your community is a long-term care facility, a new retirement home, or the old neighborhood, you can adapt them to fit your situation.

Scrapbooks

1. Assuming you could partnership with a local school where kids would visit the elderly and the elderly would go to the school, discuss the following:
   a. How would you have the young people and the old people interact?
   b. What benefits would you see for the young people from such a visit?
   c. How do you think the old people would benefit from such a visit?
   d. What programs could you envision the elderly offering to a classroom of kids? Discuss educational possibilities they could offer.

2. Make a list of all the various groups that meet within your community (scouting, quilting clubs, coin/stamp collectors, chess clubs, gourmet/cooking clubs, collectors of any kind, etc.). Once you have the list, discuss the following:
   a. What benefits could *each* of these groups or

/organizations have by associating more with the elderly?

b. Are there benefits to caretakers from working with such groups? What are they?

c. Who would schedule the programs for such groups? (In a facility consider creating a task force instead of giving it all to the Activity Department.)

d. Ask the caregivers you know who are collectors (of any kind) to display their collections. What benefits would this bring to the elderly and the caregivers?

3. If you are in a facility, what kind of community outreach do you have? Brainstorm what your facility and staff could offer to the community? Ask *each* department to do this. What benefits are there in this for the community? For your staff?

4. Part of Martin's treasures were his scrapbooks. Consider helping the elderly make a scrapbook. How could the families be involved? What kinds of things could be in the scrapbook that would help caretakers relate to the elderly?

5. Discuss the following idea: Have caregivers make their own scrapbook for the people they care for to look at so they can get to know them better.

a. Does knowing one another better improve relationships? Discuss.

b. If caregivers made up a personal scrapbook, what kinds of things do you think would be interesting for the elderly?

c. Discuss the benefits for the elderly of having caregivers' scrapbooks to look at.

6. Martin's scrapbook documented all the things of his life that he considered important. Do your caregivers know the important and meaningful events in the lives of the people they care for? If they did, in what ways would that be helpful to the caregiv-

ers? How could this be done while still respecting the elderly's rights and privacy issues?

Uniquely Unique

1. Bessie always cared about being dressed nicely. For her, it was a question of maintaining her dignity. With that in mind:
    a. Brainstorm and come up with a list of rights for the elderly that affirm their right to dignity (e.g., the right to be dressed nicely).
    b. Pick out the five most important dignity issues you have listed in la. Select teams of two and give them each *one* of the five. Tell them to observe for a period of time (perhaps a week) how your community as a whole respects that one particular dignity issue. At the end of the time period, have the teams report back to the entire group and report their observations.
    c. Of the five listed in 1b, rank them in terms of how well your community does at respecting the dignity of the elderly. Celebrate what you do well, and then discuss how you can improve upon the ones that you fall short on.

2. Training caregivers to be sensitive to dignity issues is important. What kind of training do your caregivers presently receive?

3. Dignity issues are not only for the elderly, but caregivers as well. Brainstorm the things you would list under the heading, Caregiver Bill of Rights for Dignity in the Workplace.
    a. Of the listing you have just made, prioritize them and select the top 5 to 10.
    b. Of the list you have prioritized, which ones are being affirmed in your community? Which ones are not?
    c. Of the ones in 3b not being affirmed, what could be done to improve upon those?

    d. Whose responsibility is it within your community to make sure staff dignity is respected?

    e. If you feel your dignity rights have been violated, what is the formal procedure to address that?

My Friend Flicka

1. In Zelma's story, there is mention about all the things residents have to deal with on a daily basis when they live in a long-term care facility. With that in mind, discuss how caregivers should handle the following situations:

    a. A resident has a stroke during mealtime. What should be done for those who were at the same table after the resident who had the stroke is taken out? What about residents at other tables who witnessed it?

    b. Two residents are involved in a verbal, heated argument. What should you do? What if you come upon residents who are physically fighting?

    c. A resident becomes verbally and/or physically abusive toward *you*. How can you handle the situation?

2. Zelma was called a role model. Have caregivers discuss what kind of role model they could be for other caregivers. What kinds of qualities would go into being a caregiver role model?

The Leprechaun

1. When Einar left the third floor, the staff had a going-away party for him. If you are in a facility, think about these questions:

    a. How are resident moves handled within your facility? Are assessments made in terms of the number of moves a resident makes within a time period? If not, who could make them and how could they be useful?

    b. In what intentional ways are potential roommates evaluated as being compatible (*before* the move is made)?

   c. If your facility has asked the resident to move to another room and he/she doesn't want to move, does he/she have the right to contest the transfer? If yes, what would be the steps the resident could take?

   d. Discuss ways in which moves within your facility can be put in the best possible light for the resident (for example, have the new room decorated with balloons and a "Welcome" sign).

2. Outside a facility, the elderly sometimes have to move, too. What are the best ways to prepare the person for a move? If the move is required because the current care situation is not working, how can the negative impact be minimized for both the person who is moving and the caretakers involved?

Heroism consists in hanging on one minute longer.

— *Norwegian Proverb*

Thanks for the Memories

Hewert has no family other than a second cousin who lives in another state. He hasn't had contact with his cousin for years. According to Hewert, he had heard through an acquaintance that the cousin, a widow, recently went to live in a nursing home. "I've gotten to the age," Hewert says matter-of-factly, "where I've outlived just about everybody I know, and those I haven't are in worse shape than I am." Though he hasn't had a visitor since he first arrived, he doesn't want sympathy. "I may be alone," he says, "but I ain't lonely. My mind is still good and I have a lot of memories. They keep me going." He pauses for a moment. "Hell, memories are all I got left."

A resident for nearly five years, Hewert is a proud person who wants to retain his dignity and independence, but is finding it increasingly more difficult because of his declining physical condition. His move into the Home happened when he loathingly admitted he could no longer care for himself. He has a number of ailments including Parkinson's disease. It is a disease he says he wouldn't wish on his worst enemy.

Within the past two years, Hewert has fallen several times trying to transfer from his wheelchair on his own. The last fall occurred six months ago when he decided that it was time for him to lie down for an afternoon nap. He had thought about putting the call light on for assistance but decided he could make the transfer himself. "Besides," he told me in a gravelly voice, "when I want to take a nap, I want to do it when I'm tired, and not have to wait for someone to answer the damn call light." However, he forgot to secure the wheelchair's locks and consequently, when he raised himself up, his wheelchair rolled back, causing him to lose his balance. Besides bruises on his arms and a cut on his forehead, unfortunately, the fall also resulted in a fractured hip. The hip took nearly a month to heal to the point where he could tolerate the pain from being transferred in and out of his wheelchair. Up until then, he had to depend upon pain medication.

It was Hewert's fractured hip as well as his declining physical condition from Parkinson's disease that led his doctor to strongly recommend a restraint belt. Such a belt is similar to that of a car seat belt, only this belt is used to prevent him from slipping out of his wheelchair. Hewert simply became too susceptible to falls. The suggestion for the restraint belt came as a last resort. The doctor told Hewert, "It's for your own good." It was obvious to the staff that without the belt, the chances were very good that Hewert would fall again since he still was so determined to be independent. They knew he would continue to try things that he should not be doing without assistance. In addition, they were also concerned that even if Hewert didn't fall trying to transfer, there was still the risk of his slipping out of the wheelchair when he dozed. Because they were concerned about his falling and reinjuring himself, the staff pleaded with him to follow the doctor's advice. After a great deal of urging and after another occasion when he nearly did slip out of his chair, Hewert finally agreed to the restraint belt.

Within a couple of weeks, however, Hewert was having second thoughts. "Hell, what's the point of living while being confined to a wheelchair and having to depend upon someone when you want to go to bed or have to go to the toilet." He paused for a long time and then pointed to his waist with a trembling finger. "And what the hell is the purpose of being strapped in all the time? That ain't living. I'd rather have the damn thing off and take the risk of falling." It didn't matter to him that he had the freedom to release himself from the belt without assistance. For Hewert, it was the just the idea of having it around him. It was symbolic of his loss of independence.

Hewert's struggle to maintain his personal dignity and independence while at the same time trying to cope with his declining physical condition is not unlike the struggle of other residents who are waging their own personal battles. Sam, for example, detests the thought of having to wear a diaper because of his incontinence. After having an accident at a social gathering, however, Sam reluctantly agreed to wear one. Close to tears one afternoon, he blurted out, "I'm so embarrassed. I'm afraid to go anywhere for fear of having an accident. It's so terrible, and I don't think people understand." To add to Sam's anguish, he smelled of urine and he knew it. "I have no control," he laments, "no control." Another resident who feels her independence and dignity eroding with age is Mary. She was at one time a ballet dancer who, in her twenties, toured in Europe. She has been confined to a wheelchair so long now that she confesses, "I have forgotten what it's even like to walk, let alone dance." Then there is Clarence. His hands are so crippled with arthritis that he can no longer play the piano as he so loved to do. Another resident, Frank, a ninety-two-year-old man residing on the third floor of the Chronic Care Center, sang for years in his church choir. Now, he can barely be understood because of a recent stroke that severely affected his speech. Finally, there is Josephine who once commanded the rapt attention of the students she taught, but now only commands the attention of the staff that clothe and feed her every day. All of these persons feel that they have lost or are losing their independence as well as their dignity.

Often a resident can become so frustrated with losing control of so many things that he or she wonders if it is worth going on. Some decide it is not and want to end their own lives. This was the case with a recently arrived resident who came to our facility because of chronic pain. He had been told by medical personnel that they could do nothing other than continue to increase the pain medication. His weakened condition confined him to bed. Only occasionally was he able to sit in a chair for short periods of time. The intense pain he was experiencing on a daily basis was controllable with medication, but only to a certain degree. The suffering was evident in his face and caused him to look even older than his seventy-nine years. I asked him toward the end of our visit if I could be of any help in any way. His unflinching reply was, "You could poison me," and then, realizing to whom he was talking, added, "I suppose you can't do that." Another resident whose body was twisted like a gnarled tree trunk echoed those sentiments when she kept asking the nursing staff to give her a pill so that she could go "to sleep." Her family, sitting in the room with her, wept as they heard her repeated request.

While Hewert has never asked for any kind of "sleeping pill," his increasing dependence upon others has caused him to admit that he is depressed. "Hell, who wouldn't be?" he says as he slowly raises his trembling hands. While he doesn't say it out loud, we both know that the tremors are symbolic of how he feels his dignity is being slowly taken away and that he has no control over what is happening. When asked what others could do that would be helpful, he answers without a moment's hesitation, "Remember who I was. Even though I'm eighty-seven and am confined to this damn chair, I once was a corporate executive and had over fifty employees under my command." He paused and takes a deep breath. When he begins again, he is pleading for understanding. "At one time I was in such good shape that even at twice their age, I could run circles around these kids who take care of me now. They can take care of my body because it's old and needs help, but I'm still me. Don't treat me as if I don't know anything."

The struggle for Hewert continues to be in his trying to maintain as much independence and dignity as possible. The challenge for us who care for Hewert and all the other residents is in what we can do or say to help them keep these important attributes that are valued and which none of us ourselves would want to lose.

New Beginnings

"If I have to do that, I'm going to commit suicide," Elizabeth declared that Tuesday afternoon at her care conference. Her daughter, sitting with her, tried to persuade her mother that what the staff was suggesting was for her own good, but got nowhere. Elizabeth was convinced that the staff had turned against her and no longer cared. In her threat, Elizabeth was not only expressing her own hurt and pain, but also wanting the staff to feel what she was feeling. With the news she had received, Elizabeth felt her life was ending and she wanted those whom she held responsible to hear her cries of fear, despair, and anger.

Care conferences are held for residents four times a year and are a mandatory state requirement. The conferences are meant to be opportunities for the resident and family to meet with staff to hear about and discuss their care. The care conference team, made up of staff from various disciplines, give an evaluation of the progress they think the resident is making in areas such as rehabilitation after a fall or activities of daily living (ADLs), including dressing and personal grooming. Reviews are made of medications, diet, and treatment of current physical problems, such as cataracts, edema, or any number of the other ailments that can come with age. The residents also have the opportunity to bring up any concerns they may have about their overall physical care as well as how they view life within the home itself.

Resident concerns often cover anything from questions about how a certain meal is prepared, to why they are not getting their baths on time, to what will be done about their next-door neighbor who has her television on too loud at night. Most of the time, care conferences are fairly routine, except, of course, when the staff has the task of informing residents of news that they know will be unwelcome. Such was the case for Elizabeth.

Elizabeth had come to her care conference that day with some apprehension that she was going to hear news she didn't want to hear. After the preliminaries were out of the way, she was informed that, because of her declining physical condition requiring more staff time and a higher level of care, the staff made the decision to recommend that she be transferred from the Board and Care section to the Chronic Care Center. Elizabeth left the meeting convinced that she had been betrayed by staff that no longer cared what happened to old people. When the staff informed her that she had the right to appeal their decision to the State, Elizabeth's only response had been her suicide declaration.

"We had no choice," a nurse said to the others after Elizabeth left. The tone in her voice revealed the frustration of having to make such a recommendation. The entire care conference team had agonized over what they had decided to recommend. They knew their decision was one that affected a person they had come to know well over a period of years. That it was the right decision and that Elizabeth's daughter was in agreement did not make it any easier for them. "That poor woman just couldn't do the things for herself she needed to do, and we gave her as much staff time as we could," a member of the team said to no one in particular as she looked around at the others who were involved in the difficult recommendation. She sighed before going on. "In fact, we've given her more than her share. I don't know if she realizes how demanding her level of care has gotten to be for the staff we have here." Another staff member piped in, "I hope once she makes the adjustment she'll understand Chronic Care can make life better for her."

The staff involved in making these decisions concerning Elizabeth and others in similar situations understand the trauma a move to Chronic Care causes for residents. They are not always sure, however, that residents realize how emotionally draining such decisions are on those charged with the responsibility of making them. In Elizabeth's case, the team documents her threat to commit suicide and assigns certain staff to follow up with one-to-one visits. They will also alert the staff in Chronic Care to whom Elizabeth's care will soon be entrusted. Having done that, they now have to put aside their emotions, since they still have three more care conferences to conduct before the afternoon is over.

That Elizabeth does not want to move is understandable when one considers that where she lives now, Board and Care, is a section within the facility where residents live with relative independence. Her room may be small but, nevertheless, it is private. Having a room to herself was a living arrangement that Elizabeth had thoroughly enjoyed from that first day she became a resident seven years earlier. Another aspect Elizabeth enjoyed was that she had her own private bathroom. "Something," of which she says, "the older one gets, the more one appreciates." The eating arrangements in Board and Care, though, are a different story. Even though Elizabeth tolerated sharing meals with others in a common dining area, she would have preferred the option of having a meal by herself every now and then. She admitted that the dining room was like an elegant restaurant but noted, "One can get tired of eating restaurant food three times a day, especially when you have to sit at a table with three other people all the time."

The eating arrangements in the Chronic Care Center, as Elizabeth well knew by talking to other residents, would be far less desirable. Although the dining area is pleasant (not so pleasant as Board and Care's in Elizabeth's opinion — certainly not like a restaurant), it has a much different ambiance. The new eating area would be closer to the kind of setting one typically expects to find in a nursing home. Certain people need to be fed by staff. It would not be uncommon to see, at some tables, a resident dozing while still holding a utensil. Most of the residents wear bibs because of frequent spills caused by unsteady hands. Every now and then, a resident may yell out at no one in particular.

The Chronic Care Center has three floors, with those needing the least care on first floor and those needing the most care, on the third floor. Elizabeth was told that she would be transferred to a room on the second floor and, if things went well with physical and occupational therapy, she would have a chance to move to the first floor. Since there are few private rooms, most rooms are shared by two residents. Elizabeth would be moving into a double room and placed on the waiting list for a private room. All the rooms, unfortunately, have the look and feel of a hospital setting with the double rooms having only a curtain dividing the two beds. Elizabeth knew that though her previous room was small, her new room would be smaller still. Worst of all, she would have to share a bathroom.

Elizabeth suspected she needed more care, but she had been determined to stay in the more independent Board and Care area. After hearing the review of her care needs, however, she privately told me that it was evident to her that such a move was necessary, although she would not admit that to the care conference team. Even though the staff told her that she had the right to appeal their decision to the State, Elizabeth said that she wouldn't be doing that. Besides, her daughter had pleaded with her to make the move.

It had been decided that Elizabeth would move to the second floor of the Chronic Care Center as soon as there was an opening. A week later after her care conference, on a Wednesday morning, she was told that she would be moving the following day. "Humph," she groused, "someone must have died." It was that evening, after dinner, when Elizabeth reminded the staff of her intention to commit suicide.

Moving from Board and Care to the Chronic Care Center is seldom an easy transition although there have been those who took it in stride. Many residents speak of those who are living in "that other place," as "those poor, unfortunate souls." Most living in Board and Care, in speaking of themselves and those living in Chronic Care, use the terms of "we" and "they." One Board and Care resident, in unabashed frankness, spoke words that probably were the thoughts of many: "I don't want to go over there. When you go there, you know it's the end. They're sending you over there to die." These words also reflect the feelings many people have about nursing homes: "They're places where you go to die." Given those kinds of sentiments, it is little wonder that Elizabeth reacted the way she did.

Five months have gone by since Elizabeth made the move and, admittedly, the first week or two was rather traumatic for her. She has, however, forgotten about being so angry with the care conference team and has not once mentioned suicide. Staff from Board and Care (including those who were part of the care conference team that recommended the move) visit Elizabeth whenever they get a chance; that is, if they can find her in her room. She has become involved in a variety of activities and has made several new friends that she absolutely adores. One of them is Dorothy, her roommate. "We have so much in common," Elizabeth says, "we can talk and talk like we have been friends for years." Elizabeth's health had declined further and she appreciates the extra care she receives. Although she is no longer able to do some of the things she could do just a few months ago, she says, "I'm so happy I'm here. They take such good care of me." Her only concern now is whether to move down to the first floor if she ever is presented with the opportunity. She isn't sure she wants to leave her room-mate.

Not all the stories of residents who make the move will have the positive ending Elizabeth's story had. However, her threat to commit suicide when told of such a move and then to have the move's outcome be so positive is not an exception. When threat-ened with change of that kind, older people do have fear and anxi-ety, especially as they come face to face with moving into a "nursing home." But they don't have to go it alone. Staff, volun-teers, and family are all key players in helping assure the person that he or she can adapt to such a change.

Elizabeth is now settled and she no longer feels the trauma of the change, but what about the members of the care conference team who were emotionally exhausted after having to make such a decision? As one member of the team commented, "It's nice to see that Elizabeth made the adjustment. We didn't know if she would. As for ourselves, we're doing okay. Taking it a day at a time." She adds after a moment of reflection, "You know, each decision like that takes a little bit out of you."

Tomorrow morning the care conference team is meeting with a man who is extremely angry about its being suggested that he should consider being transferred over to the Chronic Care Center. He isn't threatening suicide, but he is threatening to tell his girl-friend to hire a lawyer. When I went in to see him, he was cussing and generally raising a racket.

"What's the problem?" I asked, as if I didn't know.

"Damn it, they (the care conference team) are out to get me. They're going to send me over to that &*/@*& place with all those old people. I sure as hell don't want to be with them. I'm getting a lawyer. I don't belong there with those people."

After failing to calm him down, I asked him how old he was. I had hopes of changing the subject.

"I'm ninety-seven," he answered and then proceeded to again tell me how angry he was, and how he was going to hate it over there with all those *old* people.

I left his room that day thinking that I certainly didn't envy the care conference team who would be meeting with him tomorrow.

In Sickness and in Health

The marriage vows Norm and his wife, Berniece, made to each other over fifty-five years ago have always been important to the two of them. On their fiftieth wedding anniversary, they celebrated the occasion by having a ceremony at the church where they were married. Witnessed by relatives, a few friends, and two members from their original wedding party, Norm and Berniece renewed their marriage vows.

There is one part of the vows, however, that has taken on special significance to Norm in recent years — the phrase, *In sickness and in health*. Norm says that Berniece would also agree that these words have added meaning now that they are both in their late seventies, and she would say so, that is, if she could speak.

Berniece is on the third floor of the Chronic Care Center. She suffered a near fatal stroke three years ago that affected her mental capacity and has left her physically helpless. Completely paralyzed on one side with no hope of recovery, Berniece is confined to a wheelchair. As for any spoken communication, she has not uttered an intelligible word since the day she had her stroke. Upon occasion, she will utter grunting sounds that, at first, gave Norm some hope that she was regaining her speech. The doctors, however, thought that the sounds probably indicated she was in some kind of discomfort, and perhaps had an upset stomach or a headache. Whether she understands you when you talk to her can only be hoped for because there is no response from her at all. She stares vacantly into space and only, at times, will follow movement with her eyes. It is difficult for her to even sit straight in her wheelchair. Often, she slumps to one side, head down, drooling from the side of her mouth. Whenever Norm is at the Home with Berniece, he is continually straightening her so that she sits upright. He also carries with him a box of tissues for wiping the corners of her mouth.

For Norm, the woman sitting lifeless in the wheelchair is a far different Berniece than he remembers. He shared with me how his wife was always so active, and scarcely had time to sit. "My wife took great pride in how she looked," he proudly says, "and she spent considerable time in her grooming. I used to get so mad at her because she took so much time. Now, I would be so happy if …" His voice trails off as he turns aside, unable to finish. As Norm reminisced about how his wife was before the stroke, I saw the pain in his eyes and heard the sorrow in his voice. He loves Berniece as much today as he did the day they got married, but he will tell you that he grieves the loss of the relationship they once had.

Norm tries to be with Berniece every day, coming to the nursing home around mid-morning and staying through the supper hour. The only days he has missed were when he himself had been sick and once for three days when his doctor practically ordered him to get away for a few days to get some rest. Norm feels it is especially important to be with his wife during the noon and supper meals because Berniece is unable to feed herself. He wants to make sure she eats the way he feels she should be eating. Although the staff would feed her and are good about doing it in a caring way, Norm prefers to do it. "I need to do it as much for myself as I do for her," he candidly admits. It's another way for him to be personally involved with his wife. He patiently tries to get her to eat, and throughout the meal, he will talk to her quietly, wiping her mouth with a napkin from time to time. At other times during the day, Norm can be seen pushing Berniece in her wheelchair around the facility. He and his wife have become familiar figures to staff throughout the many sections of the Home. "It's important," Norm explains, "to get my wife away from her room and the third floor. Believe me, she receives good care by the staff. It's just that she needs a change every now and then. Maybe different scenery will stimulate her." There is a note of hope in his voice as he shares that last thought.

On some afternoons one can find Norm and Berniece in the lounge area on the first floor in the Chronic Care Center. Norm watches people come and go, greeting those whom he has gotten to know and who, like himself, have a spouse living at the Home. Upon other occasions, Norm will take his wife to the lobby area of the Assisted Living Building; that building is connected to the Chronic Care Center by a corridor. Twice a week a resident comes to play the old favorites on the grand piano in the Assisted Living lobby. Norm will wheel Berniece to a favorite spot near the piano, pull up a chair next to her wheelchair, and put his arm around her while holding her hand with his free hand. Berniece, who rarely responds to Norm's presence, often falls asleep. According to Norm, his wife will occasionally respond to the music by blinking her eyes. Sometimes, when a song is played that was a favorite of Berniece's, she will move her head toward the piano. Norm sighs and says about his wife's response to the music, "At least, it's something."

Not well himself, Norm is not sure how much longer he will be able to spend this much daily time with Berniece. He had by-pass surgery last year and recently had an ambulance ride to the hospital because of chest pains. The doctors diagnosed it as an angina attack, but Norm wonders what it would be the next time. "I'm living on borrowed time," he says, reflecting upon the days he spent in the hospital and the thoughts that went through his mind while lying in the hospital bed. "I realized how fragile life is." He told me that his concern was not about himself, but rather about his wife. They had one daughter who, tragically, was killed in an automobile accident over twenty years ago. Their daughter was only in her late thirties. "I've had two terrible things happen in my life," Norm says. "The first was when our daughter was killed. The second was when my wife had her stroke." Without any close relatives, Norm knows that if he were not able to see her, his wife would be alone. He says that he sometimes wakes up in the middle of the night and thinks about Berniece. The only thing that enables him to go back to sleep is knowing that there are staff at the Home who are caring for his wife when he is not there. He will tell you that with the health problems he and his wife have, he hopes Berniece dies first.

Speaking candidly, Norm will tell you that he envies another man whose wife is also on the third floor and who is nearly in as bad shape as Berniece. He envies him because this man's wife will, upon some occasions, utter a word or two that shows she seems to be aware of her surroundings and that her husband is with her. I was with this man and his wife one Christmas, and I said to the two of them, "Have a Merry Christmas." To my surprise, his wife responded by saying, "Merry Christmas to you also." The husband was so pleased because he had not heard his wife say anything for nearly two months. He told Norm and me a couple of days later, "Hearing her say those words was the best Christmas present ever." Norm smiled and said that he was happy for him. I could see the anguish in his eyes, however, as he no doubt wished that Berniece could have acknowledged his presence on Christmas.

Norm represents a number of spouses who have had to watch their wives or husbands sit in a wheelchair or lie in a bed day after day. "Growing old together as a couple is not always like the advertisements portrayed on television," Norm says. He and others like him in similar circumstances, however, are renewing their marriage vows day by day, especially that part that says "in sickness and in health."

Legacies

Margaret was late for her own funeral.

The service that cold afternoon in January was to start at one-thirty. The chapel at the nursing home was ready. The choir was ready. The organist was ready. The chaplain was ready. The family and friends were ready. Margaret, however, was not. After I conferred with the family, it was decided that if Margaret didn't arrive by two o'clock, we would begin without her. Perhaps a word of explanation is in order before describing any further events of that afternoon.

Margaret had lived at the nursing home for nearly fifteen years. After a chest cold had suddenly taken a turn for the worse, Margaret developed pneumonia. She died within a couple of weeks. Margaret was two months away from her ninety-second birthday when she slipped away peacefully during the early morning hours. As she had requested, the family had her body cremated. Her ashes were to be brought to the chapel for the service. This responsibility had been taken on by one of her sons who had flown in from another part of the country. Driving to the chapel, however, the son came upon a detour. After taking a wrong turn on the unfamiliar road, he became hopelessly lost. Eventually, he found himself on the right road again only to get tied up in a traffic jam. When he finally arrived at the chapel, he hurried in, and being a little chagrined, announced with a sheepish smile to the waiting grandchildren and other members of the family. "I took Grandma for a ride." His words were received with laughter, and heads nodding knowingly that this was fitting for Margaret since one could usually expect the unexpected from her.

Going for a ride and being late for her funeral would have tickled Margaret and, no doubt, she would have said to those who had patiently waited, *Oh, you were such dears to wait for me. I love you all for being so nice,* and parenthetically, she would have added, *Let's get this show on the road now. There's no time to waste.* In all the years she was a resident, Margaret was never the type to be content just to sit in a rocking chair and rock away the time.

When Margaret first arrived at the Home, she moved into Board and Care, an area of the nursing home where residents live more independently and do not require the level of care required by those residing in the Chronic Care Center. From the moment she moved in, Margaret resolved to live life in her new home to the fullest every minute of every day. She was especially determined to be as independent as she possibly could. The various physical ailments she developed over the years may have slowed her activity, but they didn't prevent her from exerting her independence. Shortly after she arrived, for example, she developed edema. The prescribed treatment for this affliction called for Margaret to stay off her feet as much as possible until the swelling went down in her ankles and legs. The nursing staff, however, had all they could do just to get her to sit in her chair for more than an hour. Often, as soon as they left her room, closing the door behind them, Margaret would be up and walking around. When told by an aide that it was for her own good to sit in a chair with her feet up, Margaret's response was, "I know I'm supposed to, but at my age, I can't afford to sit around. Besides," she asked, "how am I supposed to go to the bathroom sitting here?"

As the years went on, Margaret's spirit of independence became even more apparent after she physically declined to the point where additional care was needed and, as a consequence, she was transferred to the Chronic Care Center. Being now confined to a wheelchair, though, didn't stop her as she quipped, "Good, at least *this* chair has wheels."

In time, Margaret became a legend among staff as they told stories about not finding her in her room and then searching the buildings to no avail. After alerting staff throughout the facility about Margaret's disappearance, her nurses would go back to Margaret's room only to discover her sitting in her wheelchair reading a magazine. "Where have you been?" they asked with exasperation. "We've looked all over for you!" Margaret would simply smile and reply nonchalantly, "No place in particular. Just around."

The determination to preserve independence was something Margaret left as a legacy for other residents to follow as well. They may not reach Margaret's "legend" status, but each of their stories serves as an example of the independence she would have applauded. Sam, as a case in point, is a resident who suffered a severe stroke, leaving him with the use of only one side of his body. He, however, displays his independence by using his one good leg to pull himself forward in his wheelchair. Not satisfied simply going up and down the corridors of the second floor in the Chronic Care Center where his room is located, he travels throughout the network of buildings that make up our facility. Many residents and staff marvel at his resolve to be as self-reliant as possible. Still another resident with the tenacity of Margaret's spirit of independence is a woman who, confined to bed, refuses to let anyone turn on her television set. For her, the remote control at her side is a symbol of independence. "I may not be able to do a lot of things anymore, but this is one thing I still can do," she proclaims with a determined look in her eye.

Margaret's desire for independence is representative of many nursing home residents who are creatively discovering how to be more independent than family or staff may think they are capable of being. All of us can be indebted to Margaret and others like her for they are role models of the independent spirit we all strive for and treasure. As we age, whether or not we should ever become residents of a nursing home, we may find ourselves encouraged as well as inspired by the stories of those who have gone before us.

Margaret's legend that grew from her way of independently doing the unexpected was enhanced that cold day in January when a bouquet of flowers arrived a half-hour after her memorial service had ended. Those gathered were having coffee and cookies. The tardy delivery brought smiles as family and friends agreed it was appropriate that the flowers arrived late. Some even thought that Margaret might have arranged it.

Questions for Reflection

These questions are meant to be catalysts, to stimulate creative thinking about ways at providing quality, holistic care for the elderly. In some instances, the reflecting may lead to new (perhaps untraditional) ways of providing care. Not all questions may apply to your situation, but *all* situations will benefit from reflecting upon them. Whether your community is a long-term care facility, a new retirement home, or the old neighborhood, you can adapt them to fit your situation.

Thanks for the Memories

1. In the story, there is a resident who keeps asking the nurses for a pill she could use to "go to sleep." While the staff response may be clear in that situation, consider how you would respond in the following situations:
   a. An elderly person tells you that he can visit with anyone he wants, whenever he wants, and wherever he wants. He says it's his right.
   b. An elderly person tells you that she doesn't want to take a certain medication because it doesn't look like her medicine, or because it upsets her stomach. She says you can't force her to take it.
   c. An elderly person tells you that he can decide when to go to bed at night and when to get up in the morning.
   d. An elderly person tells you that another staff person made an inappropriate sexual advance (this person has a history of making such claims).
   e. An elderly person complains about the food being cold and wants to send it back to be reheated, claiming it's her right (she does this 2 or 3 times each week).
   f. An elderly person tells you that he is thinking about committing suicide, but asks you to promise not to tell anyone.
   g. An elderly person demands to see her medical records.

2. How would the situations in question 1 be different if the person involved were not elderly? Or is there a difference?

3. In what ways are your caregivers trained about the rights of the elderly? Who gives that training? How often is it given?
   a. If you are in a facility, are resident rights posted? If so, where? If not, why not?
   b. Who is responsible for making sure the rights of the elderly are being honored?

4. Hewert's struggle for dignity included trying to be as independent as possible. What happens when a person's independence causes more work for staff, e.g., the person wants to take therapy at a certain time to avoid conflicts with his favorite television program?

New Beginnings

1. What policies and procedures do you have in place for caregivers to follow when a person is considered suicidal?

2. In the story, Elizabeth is faced with moving from one part of the facility to another part. She expressed several concerns. Considering similar situations within your community, reflect upon the following:
   a. List all the concerns a person might have in making a move (even if it is making a move to another room in the same section of a facility).
   b. From the list of 2a, pick the top three concerns the elderly usually have. Evaluate how well you do in reducing the anxiety level of each person when it comes to these concerns.
   c. What could be done that *isn't* being done to make the move as easy a transition as possible? (If not sure, survey the elderly and/or their families and ask them: What could we have done to make this move easier?

3. The story refers to the stress often placed on care conference teams. Care conferences are required in long-term care facilities; similar processes, although less formal, occur whenever changes in care are discussed. With that in mind:
   a. What are the three major stressors care conference teams generally experience?
   b. What could be done by your community to help reduce such stress? (If you cannot think of anything, ask members of the care conference team.)

In Sickness and in Health

1. The story refers to Norm's wife who, because of a severe stroke, was severely physically and mentally impaired. Norm understands the implications of lack of communication for his relationship with his wife. Reflect upon the following questions as they deal with communication between caregivers.
    a. Define what *good* communications between caregivers would be in your community?
    b. Do you feel that communications among your caregivers is good? Why or why not?
    c. List things that work *against* the communication process in your community.
    d. From 1c, select the top 3, and discuss concrete ways that your community might work at improving them.

2. List all the ways communication is done in your community. Which are the most effective? Why are they effective?

3. Discuss whether your community has a communication systems network. If so, diagram it out.

4. It will be said that communication is everyone's job. Talk about that in terms of your particular position within the community.
    a. What kinds of things do you do that would be important for others to know about?
    b. How do *you* communicate with those others in 4a?
    c. How might you improve communication between family members and caregivers? If not sure, ask the people you need to communicate with.

5. Norm, as a family member of a resident, spends most of his time at the nursing home. Many relatives and friends spend a great deal of time with loved ones in facilities. With such individuals in mind, reflect upon the following:

a. In what intentional ways do the caregivers seek to get to know the family members who are there on a regular basis?
b. Are there activities that family members could be invited to join? If not, what benefits might be gained for them if they were invited? How might staff benefit from family members being present?
c. Discuss the pros and cons of inviting family members to help out with activities, or doing meal times, etc. If they were willing, who would benefit and in what ways? How would they be trained? Supervised?
d. How can the community, as a whole, help support people like Norm who choose to spend their time with a loved one?

Legacies

1. Margaret's story is about having a memorial held where she was a resident. What are your feelings about a facility having memorials/funerals on site?

2. If you allow memorials/funerals to be held at a facility, should you allow the casket? Why or why not?

3. If you do not allow caskets at a facility you are involved with, discuss whether that policy needs to be re-evaluated. What would be the benefits of allowing caskets to residents, families, *and* staff?

Heaven has many cracks through which God can see.

— Russian Proverb

The Sailing Ship

"I've been dreaming about death for the past three weeks," Mavis told me one morning as she sat in my office. She searched my face for any reaction and as if she had anticipated the question I was about to ask, went on to explain, "It's not a fearful feeling, but more like I'm at peace. I have tears when I wake up, but do you know something?" As she paused, her face took on an expression of serenity. "They're tears of joy. That's possible, isn't it?"

"Yes," I replied, being aware of the overwhelming peace I was observing in this woman, "it's possible." When she smiled in response, I felt her sense of peace touching me.

In my work as a chaplain I have known many residents over the years who were not afraid of death and, as an expression of their spirituality, said they were looking forward to "going home." Many of them had asked me to offer a prayer that God might take them home soon because they felt they had lived long enough. I recall asking a woman who was in her early nineties if she was planning to live to be 100. "Goodness gracious, no," she had replied. "I had wanted the Lord to take me when I was ninety. I've lived too long as it is." Although other residents had not spoken of the tears of joy as Mavis had, her experience was in keeping with the prevalent attitude of many of her peers when it comes to the topic of death.

Mavis had appeared at the open door to my office that morning and quietly asked if I had a minute to talk with her about some dreams she had been having. I asked her to come in and sit down. The minute stretched into twenty, but I didn't mind because it turned out to be one of those special opportunities where I have the privilege of listening to another share her most intimate thoughts and feelings about life and death. Mavis' spirituality was reflected in the ideas she shared. She described them in a way in which many of the other residents have identified, as she talked about traveling the last part of her journey through life. There are, of course, residents who will inform you they have no formal ties to religion. However, these same residents will talk about believing in a power greater than themselves. An example is Sherman who, at age eighty-nine, said he had never been much of a religious person. Yet, when asked if he believed in God, he replied, "Well, I reckon I do. You gotta believe in something beyond this life, don't ya?" Sherman might not be able to identify with Mavis' formal religious upbringing, but the two of them would find common ground in the belief that there is something beyond death.

"Chaplain, I'm not afraid of death," Mavis told me. I know where I'm going." Her words were a statement of her spirituality, and the calmness in which she uttered them reflected her inner peace. There was no doubt in my mind that her tears were truly tears of joy, and I wondered how many people would understand that a person could have tears of joy upon waking up after having dreams about death. Just before Mavis left, she laughed and said, "I almost forgot to tell you the reason I stopped to talk. I wanted to share with you what my favorite Bible passage is. I just want you to remember it for later on."

"I will," I replied, and jotted it down on a card with her name on it. We both knew why she wanted me to know; no further explanation was necessary. Coming to see me was simply her way of getting things in order to prepare for that time when, as she told me that day, "My tired heart will finally be at rest." Mavis, like many of the residents, wished to have many of the funeral arrangements settled in advance so that there would be less of a burden upon family members.

The average age of the 450 residents living at our facility is in the mid-eighties. Mavis, in her early seventies, was younger than the average age. She, unfortunately, was above average in terms of her medical problems. In the past year her high blood pressure, once kept under control by medication, had played havoc with her system. She had made three trips by ambulance to a nearby hospital in the past two months. The doctors had informed her that her heart was tired and while surgery was possible, it would be very risky for her age. It would be so risky that one heart surgeon decided he would not attempt it. Another surgeon said he would, but spent nearly an hour talking with her about the things that could go wrong. This doctor had informed Mavis that the chance of her survival after surgery, given her age and other medical problems, was less than thirty percent. That was providing, however, she didn't die on the operating table, which he felt was an even greater danger. After weighing both options and talking it over with her family, Mavis decided not to have the surgery and to allow "nature to take its course." She told me two days after she had made her decision, "My body is just getting worn out, and that's what happens when you get old. It's part of life and you've got to accept it."

During the years in which I have had the opportunity to share in the lives of the elderly, hundreds of those experiences have been with residents and their families in the area of death and dying. I have had the privilege of sharing some very touching moments as, for example, the time when I was present as a son sat by his mother's bedside and held her hand. His mother, Winnifred, was dying and she knew it, but she was more concerned about her son. She had told me previously that the only thing she worried about when she died was how hard it would be on her son. The son, although nearly overcome with grief, was more concerned about his mother. Being in the room with the two of them, I was deeply moved by their love for each other.

The experience with Winnifred and her son was quite in sharp contrast to one with Burton, an elderly resident who didn't want his family to be present when he died. When I asked him what could I do for him, he told me, "Nothing." He was in such terrible pain that he welcomed death. Burton had come into the facility with terminal bone cancer and, despite medication, he was in constant pain; sometimes the pain was more than he thought anybody should have to bear. He knew that there was no hope and it was just a matter of time. "I'd just as soon get this over with," he said. For him, death would release him.

Mavis died two months after that visit in my office when she shared with me her dreams about death and waking up with tears of joy. Up until the last week of her death, she came down to our chapel on a daily basis. She told me that she sat in the chapel praying, thinking about the time ahead, and remembering family and friends who had died over the years. "I'll be happy to see them again," she said.

A nurse who was with Mavis when she died reported to me that Mavis sat up in bed as if reaching for someone who was there in the room, and when she lay back down, she was smiling. The nurse said that she died a few minutes later.

Mavis reminded me of a woman who once came to see me to ask about what she should do; she was traveling to another state to see her brother who was dying of cancer and had asked to see her. The woman wondered how to act and what to talk about when she entered her brother's hospital room. She was afraid to do or say the wrong thing. I told her to be natural and let her inner feelings speak for her. "More than likely," I said, "your brother will want to talk about his death." I told her that she should not be afraid of crying in front of him and that she should say the things she wanted and needed to say for closure. Two weeks later this woman called to tell me that, "It was a beautiful experience. We cried together," she said. "We laughed together. My brother died the second day of my visit. I was with him. It was sad, of course, but it was a beautiful death," she said and then added, "Many of my friends look at me strangely when I tell them about what a beautiful experience it was. I don't think they understand."

Perhaps many people would not understand. That is unfortunate, but I know of one who would have; her name was Mavis. There is a particular piece of writing by Henry van Dyke that she so enjoyed that, she said, expressed her feelings about dying. In her memory, I share it:

> *I am standing on a seashore. A ship at my side spreads her white sails to the morning breeze and starts for the ocean blue. She is an object of beauty and strength, and I stand and watch her until at length she hangs like a speck of white cloud just where the sea and sky come down to meet each other. Then someone at my side says, "There,*

she is gone."

Gone where? Gone from my sight, that is all. She is just as large in mast and hull and spar as she was when she left my side, and just as able to bear her load of living weights to its place of destination. Her diminished size is in me, not in her, and just at the moment when someone says, "There she is gone," on that distant shore there are other eyes watching for her coming and other voices ready to take up the glad shout, "There she comes," and such is dying.

Amazing Grace

Giving the Sacrament of Holy Communion is a high point of any minister's work. It is a holy and sacred moment, but I have to admit, there are times when I'm administrating the Sacrament that I have trouble keeping a straight face. Ironically, these are also the very moments when I am most challenged to review my theology and understanding of God's grace.

Besides offering communion the first Sunday of every month in the chapel, we also offer it once a month in a group setting on each of the three floors of the Chronic Care Center. It was in this group setting that I encountered Ed, one of the first residents to receive communion. As I moved on after service, he kept hollering, "Hey! Hey!" at me, obviously to regain my attention. I wondered if perhaps he was in some kind of physical discomfort, so I went back to him and asked what he needed. Looking me straight in the eye, he slammed his little plastic communion cup on the table and bellowed, "Fill it up again!"

As with many of the residents on the third floor, Ed suffers from dementia, and like the others, he can get quite confused and disoriented. The question I'm forced to wrestle with is the validity of communion for someone like Ed who does not always seem to understand what is happening. There are other residents who fall asleep during the service while some just look at the communion wafer as if it were a foreign object that they have never seen before. Of course, there are residents who have dementia who fully participate and understand clearly that they are being given the Sacrament. But what about those like Ed? Their situation was never covered by any of the professors of theology in seminary. In class we may have pondered the miracles recorded in the pages of the Bible, discussed how apocalyptic literature might be interpreted, studied the formation and theology of the church in the first century, but we never considered how our theology might deal with circumstances such as Ed's.

I have decided that if I am going to err, I will err on the side of God's grace. Ed and others like him are people who in earlier days were connected with a church and certainly participated in communion on a regular basis. Many of them were quite involved in their churches and held positions of leadership. Some of them taught young people in Sunday school and no doubt frequently talked about the importance of communion. Others may have baked the bread used, or prepared the communion trays, or even assisted in the distribution. To withhold communion from people who suffer dementia on the basis that they do not understand, does not, in my opinion, do justice to God's grace.

I would like to share with you some of the questions I struggled (and continue to struggle) with: Are there not times when we must rely solely on God's grace and trust it to reach people in ways beyond our awareness? Is there a need for us to get in touch with our common humanity so that we might be open in discovering how working with people like Ed can enhance our own understanding of God? Are we willing to approach circumstances like Ed's and be open to perhaps meeting God on new and holy grounds? How do we know when our approach is too dogmatic? Is it possible that our consciousness of spirituality could be raised through encounters with those who have dementia? Can God speak to us through a person like Ed? More importantly, if God is speaking to us through someone like Ed, what are we being told? And, are we really listening? Giving communion in a nursing home will continue to challenge me to re-examine my theology, and that is as it should be. Just the other day, for example, I was explaining to a new resident who was a Methodist that I was the chaplain, a Lutheran minister, and that we offer communion once a month in the chapel. I then said, "I offer it once a month on the floor as well." Of course, I meant that we offer communion once a month in a group setting on each of the three floors of the Chronic Care Center besides having it in the chapel. As soon as I said we offer it on the floor, however, I knew something was not right; she gave me a strange look, glanced down at the floor, and replied quietly, "Oh, I'm a Methodist. I don't think we do that."

I don't think Lutherans do it either but then again, as I said, doing this work continually challenges me to review my theology.

Never a Wrong Number

Beverly Mae is a resident at a nursing home, but not at the one where I work as a chaplain. She is, however, always welcome to come and live at ours. For that matter, I believe any nursing home would love to have her as a resident. I feel confident in saying that because, in my opinion, Beverly Mae is an excellent representative of those within her age group. She exemplifies the characteristics of many of our senior citizens with her humor, faith, and enduring spirit. She has such an outgoing personality that she would be a natural spokesperson for any organization that has as its goal to educate the general public as to the vitality and vigor of the over sixty-five age group. If you want a role model to follow as you approach your later years, I believe she would be an ideal one.

With everything I have said about Beverly Mae, you may think that I have known her for a long time to characterize her in such a positive way. The truth of the matter is that I have never met her. I have only talked with her on the telephone for a few brief moments. I don't even know her real name. She didn't tell me. I call her Beverly Mae only because she reminded me of a woman with that name who was a member of the small country church I served years ago.

The first time I met the real Beverly Mae was on a hot, humid summer day in July. Others had told me that she was a person I would want to get to know, but they didn't tell me why.

"You'll find out," those who knew her said. My curiosity piqued, I decided to pay her a visit. I drove to the farmhouse where Beverly Mae lived with her daughter and her daughter's family. When no one answered my knocking at the front door, I went around to the back, hoping to find someone. I did. There was a woman in an ankle-length dress and a weathered straw hat. She was down on her hands and knees pulling weeds from the garden. She was singing softly to herself. At first, I thought it was the daughter, but soon learned to my surprise that it was Beverly Mae. As I was to discover in the many visits we were to have, she was one of the liveliest personalities I had ever had the pleasure to know. My first clue of her zest for life was when I told her that day I first met her that I thought it seemed quite hot to be working in the garden. She looked up at me and replied, "My mother used to work in her garden until she was nearly 102 years old. I'm only ninety-four."

Getting back now to the woman I first mentioned; the one to whom I gave the name of Beverly Mae, and said that I talked with her only on the phone. It was a Friday evening when "Beverly Mae" called. That was the first time I had ever talked with this woman, and I'm sure it was for less than two minutes. She had dialed the wrong number. From the short telephone conversation I had with her, I realized she and the real Beverly Mae could have been identical twins because they both possessed such vitality for life.

On the evening of the phone call, my wife was watching television in the bedroom. I was downstairs working on a project. When the phone rang, both my wife and I answered, picking up different extensions. "Hello," we both said.

"Hello," a cheery voice said, "this is your mother."

"I'm sorry," my wife replied as I listened in on the extension, "but you must have the wrong number. My mother is dead. She died ten years ago."

"Oh, I'm so sorry," the woman said in a tone that indicated she felt terribly upset over initially having made such a remark.

"Wait a minute," I pleaded, thinking she was going to hang up. I had a hunch about the caller that I wanted to test out. Besides, I didn't want her to feel so bad. "Where are you calling from?" I asked in a tone of voice that I hoped sounded upbeat and light-hearted.

"I am calling from _____" She named a nursing home in the area whose name I immediately recognized. It confirmed my suspicion that the caller was someone in her later years.

I wanted to say something that would put her more at ease since I suspected she was still feeling bad about saying, "This is your mother" to someone whose mother had died. Taking a chance that the caller would catch the humorous lilt in my voice, I said, "Oh, I thought you were calling from heaven."

The caller laughed and without a moment's hesitation replied in a lighthearted tone of voice, "Oh, I wish I were."

We exchanged a few more pleasantries, and then I hung up my extension while my wife and she talked for another minute. Afterwards, my wife said the woman sounded nice but kept apologizing for dialing the wrong number. We smiled about the phone call and the woman's retort to my inquiry. As I thought about her retort, I realized that it was just another example of the wit, humor, and faith one can expect to find among those who reside in a nursing home.

If by chance your phone should ring tonight and a voice you don't recognize says, "This is your mother," don't hang up; it just might be *Beverly Mae*. If it is, you're in for a delightful treat even if it is the wrong number.

Believing is Seeing

"You're going to think I'm crazy," Claire said to me just as I was making myself comfortable in one of the chairs in her room.

Claire was sitting opposite me, not more than three feet away, in her favorite chair, a light blue recliner. The chair was designed to provide instant comfort and relaxation. She, however, was far from relaxed as she sat perched on its edge waiting for my reply. Staff had told me that Claire had made a request to talk with me. I had no idea what it was about, but her opening statement certainly got my attention.

"I won't think you're crazy," I replied, fairly confident that I had heard just about everything in over twenty-five years of ministry, and very little now, I thought, would surprise me. I wanted to tell her to just lean back and relax, to get her money's worth out of the chair; pull up the handle and get comfortable.

"Do you remember my son, John, who died two years ago?" Claire asked. "He was my oldest."

"I vaguely remember your talking about him," I replied. I was thinking that this might be a grief counseling situation since two years is not very long to be still grieving over the death of a child, even when that child was a retired business man in his early seventies. Claire, like most her age, never thought she would outlive her children, and more than once had commented to staff how life is so unfair. She isn't the only resident who has had that unfortunate experience. It happens more often than people realize and can be devastating to the elderly parent. I thought about that as I asked Claire, "Did I ever meet your son?"

"I don't think so," she replied. "He lived too far away and hadn't been in good health over the past few years." Claire paused and looked aside for a moment. "He never made it here to visit me but we talked on the telephone twice a week. John was very good about calling. He was a good boy. You see, he was my first-born and we were very close." She paused again, and by the look on her face, I sensed that she was experiencing an unspoken memory about her son. That quickly passed, however, as she leaned forward even further in her chair, so much so, I was concerned she might accidentally tumble forward out of it. "It was my son, John, who found my glasses this morning. Do you think that's crazy?"

"Well," I began and then stopped to clear my throat, "I have to admit that's a little out of the ordinary." I hoped that the sense of surprise I was feeling was not too obvious on my face, and now I felt myself leaning forward in my chair. "Tell me more," I said, hoping that would buy me a little more time to figure out what I was getting myself into here.

"You know I wear glasses and I'm always putting them down someplace," Claire said. I nodded my head to let her know I was following her. "The other day I misplaced them," she continued. "I just couldn't find them. My daughter was visiting yesterday and she helped me look. Even one of the aides came in to help us look. The three of us looked the whole room over and we found nothing. I had to go down to the dining room last night without my glasses," she exclaimed. "We just couldn't find them."

As I sat there listening, I glanced around her room. There was a television sitting on a small cabinet in one corner; a twin bed with two large satin pillows; a teddy bear with *Grandma* embroidered on its tummy, lying against the bed pillows, its eyes staring up at the ceiling; the two chairs Claire and I were sitting on; a third chair with magazines stacked upon it standing alongside a writing desk; knick-knacks and so forth. It was the usual furniture and items one would find in a resident's room. Although a little cluttered, the room would not have taken three people very long to conduct a thorough search, and that would include searching the small closet.

As I continued to look around the room, I realized that there were not too many places to misplace an item, even something as small as a pair of glasses.

"This morning my glasses were still missing," Claire said, "and I was getting more and more anxious. I just didn't know what I was going to do." She paused to take the kind of deep breath people take when they know they're about to make an announcement that will be quite dramatic to the hearers. "Then, I felt the presence of John, and I asked him if he would help me find my glasses." Claire looked at me for a response, but I just nodded my head to let her know she had my attention. "Well," she continued, "about twenty minutes went by, and as I was dusting off the desk, something made me turn around. It was like an inner voice told me to look under the magazine by the telephone. And, Chaplain, do you know what?"

"I can only guess," I replied quietly.

"I picked up that magazine, and there were my glasses. I was so happy. As I put them on, I could feel the presence of my son in the room. I knew then that John had helped me find my glasses." Having finished her story, Claire finally leaned back in her chair, closed her eyes for a moment, and then looked at me. "Do you think this sounds crazy?"

"No," I replied truthfully. As I sat there, I thought about other such experiences. A month earlier, one of the nurses told me about what a resident named Ruth had seen the morning of the day she died. Ruth had told this nurse that something made her look up and when she did, she had seen four young girls floating above her head. Ruth said this happened right after breakfast as she sat in her wheelchair watching people go by in the hallway. She had described the girls as being very beautiful and said that they made her feel so peaceful. That afternoon, Ruth died unexpectedly. The nurse mentioned the story to me because she wondered if perhaps those four young girls were angels who had come to take Ruth home.

Another resident told me about the time when he was so seriously ill that everybody, including himself, thought he was not going to last through the night. "You're not going to believe this," he said, and then went on to tell me that at some point during the night, a person bathed in light appeared at the end of his bed. "The person didn't say anything, but just stood there for a long time. The next morning I felt better and ever since, I've not been afraid of death anymore."

Finally, there was the woman who told me of the untimely death of her mother and how she had cried herself to sleep every night until, one evening, she saw her mother smiling and sitting in the rocking chair in her room. After that, this woman said she was able to sleep peacefully.

Claire and I talked for some time. After sharing a few of the experiences people had related to me that were similar to what Claire had experienced with her son, she felt better, knowing that I didn't think she was crazy.

Quite a few months have passed since the afternoon Claire told me the story about how her deceased son helped her to find her glasses. Yesterday, I walked past her room and her door was open. I noticed that she was sitting in her favorite chair, leaning back with her feet up on the footrest. She, however, didn't have her glasses on. I hoped that she hadn't lost them again, but then I remembered the day she told me, "You're going to think I'm crazy." As I passed her room, I smiled. I wasn't worried about her finding her glasses, and I knew she wasn't crazy.

He's Lying Again

Ernie is not exactly a member of the Pastoral Care Unit, but he is in many ways as much a part of the daily life and ministry at the nursing home as the chaplain. He stands in front of my office day after day greeting people, letting them know of the chaplain's availability by wearing a sign around his neck. The sign reads on one side: The Chaplain is In. Turn the sign over and it reads: The Chaplain is Out. People occasionally poke their heads in to let me know the sign says I am out when, actually, they see me sitting at my desk. My stock answer is, "Ernie is lying again!"

Before you begin to really wonder about Ernie, let me tell you something more about him. Ernie is a large furry puppet that I use in my work. He's supposed to be a dog but has also been thought of as a cat, a bear, even a monkey. His legs are fastened around my waist and one paw is tucked into my shirt collar behind my neck. His other paw is attached to a stick that I operate with my left hand while my right hand and arm go up through his body to move his mouth. Ernie is amazingly lifelike and has been mistaken for being real by both residents and staff. More than once, I have startled another staff member by coming around a corner with Ernie. I frequently have to tell new residents that Ernie is just a puppet. He's really more than that, though, because Ernie talks to people, and they enjoy visiting with him.

Ernie became a part of the chaplain's staff when I decided to learn ventriloquism as a way of trying some unique approaches to ministry in my work at the nursing home. I had interviewed a Catholic nun who had used this approach in working with hospital patients, including those who were terminally ill. I was encouraged by her success and that of others I read about in various kinds of settings, as, for example, the police officer who uses a ventriloquism figure as he walks the streets in a tough neighborhood.

The first time Ernie made his appearance, I was a bit apprehensive about how the residents might react. My primary concern was that they might think that it was silly and childish. My fears were unfounded because Ernie proved to be an immediate hit with both residents and staff.

Ernie talks to the residents and cozies up to them. In return, he is hugged, kissed, and stroked. One resident insisted that he sit on her lap because she loved him so much. She would ask about him when I didn't bring him around and always made me promise to greet him for her. When she was dying, Ernie visited her at her request. Although she couldn't speak and was in much discomfort, she smiled when she saw Ernie. Her family told me later how often their mother had talked about Ernie.

Another resident tells me every day to bring "the animal." I believe she would just as soon see Ernie as she would the chaplain. One day when she didn't want to get up from bed to come to lunch, Ernie and I went in to see how she was doing. As soon as she saw Ernie, she brightened up, and at his suggestion decided to come out to eat. He has become so much a part of many lives that I am often asked, "Where's Ernie?" when I don't take him around. There are a few residents who very seldom communicate with anyone, but when Ernie is present, they will talk to him. The staff has been very supportive and has told me more than once how seeing Ernie brightened up their day as well.

Ernie, I think, is popular with the residents for two reasons: the first is that he is symbolic of all the dogs or cats they have had in their lives. He represents those pets that residents could not bring with them when they entered the nursing home. No wonder he is petted, hugged, and squeezed. The second reason for his popularity is because he's so accepting of the residents. He's not afraid to be touched by them, or to lay his head on a shoulder, or to tell them a joke, or to laugh at one of their funny stories. They have fun with him. Ernie lets them enjoy their own sense of humor and gives them the freedom to express it. They know he's not real, but he's real enough to care about them and to bring some gaiety into their lives.

The residents, like any of us, need to have some fun and enjoyment. Ernie does that for them and, as long as he does, he will be part of the Pastoral Care team. It has been said that God acts in mysterious and wondrous ways to touch the lives of people. One of the ways I have witnessed the grace of God is through a furry puppet that stands out in front of my office.

Moonshine Saved My Life

"Moonshine saved my life," Mille announced to me after a glass of champagne was set down in front of her. Hearing the conviction in her voice, I had a hunch that the dinner conversation with this spunky eighty-year-old grandmother might prove to be interesting. Not all of my hunches pay off, but this one did — and with dividends, especially when Mille recounted the story of how her life was saved.

Mille, her daughter, her daughter's husband, and I were sitting at a table in the kitchen-dining room area of her granddaughter's house. We had just toasted the new bride (Mille's granddaughter) and groom who had been married within the hour.

Even though Mille admitted having slowed down over the years, her personality was more alive and spunky than many half her age. She wasn't at the point, however, where she had to begin thinking about moving into a nursing home. If that day ever came, though, Mille could apply at the one I work at. I certainly would vouch for her since, in my opinion, Mille would fit right in with the already colorful cast of *characters* we have living at the Home. With her down-to-earth personality, Mille would charm the staff and other residents. She would have no trouble getting to know others or developing new friendships. And, as a great storyteller, Mille could hold her own with the best of the other residents who are always competing with each other as to which one has the best yarn to spin.

"The moonshine came from my husband's still," Mille said. "It was hard times in the '30s. Everybody had their own still." She paused to take a sip of her champagne. "My husband made the moonshine to sell," she explained as she put her glass down. "It was a way to make a little extra money. Of course, you always made enough moonshine to keep some for yourself." She offered a half knowing smile. "We put what we kept in quart jars and stored the jars in the back of the pantry. Away from prying eyes. You know what I mean?"

"I think so," I replied.

"We lived in a small house with eight children. I was pregnant with my ninth, which was due any day." She looked at me quizzically. "Can you imagine having to look after eight small kids by yourself and being pregnant at the same time?"

I shook my head, no, and then asked, "Where was your husband?"

"Oh, I forgot to tell you," she said. "My husband was in jail." If Mille was in any way embarrassed about that fact, she didn't show it. "He was completing a six-month sentence for making moonshine."

"And you managed all by yourself?" I shook my head in disbelief. "I just can't imagine that."

"Now that I think back, neither can I," Mille replied with a chuckle. "I don't know how I did it, but the good Lord must have been watching over me." She smiled at me and I simply nodded. "You know, we didn't have any indoor plumbing in those days and the house was so small that the kids had to sleep two and three to a bed. We had two rooms upstairs, and a dirt floor for a basement."

Mille's daughter spoke up. "Tell him about the water."

"We had to pump our own water," Mille explained. "The well was out in back. I made several trips each day to get water. It seemed like all I did every day was pump water and cook, pump water and wash clothes, pump water and give baths, pump water and do the dishes."

By now I was so wrapped up in this part of the story that I had forgotten about the moonshine saving her life. "Mille, and you were pregnant. Wow!"

"Yup, I was expecting her." Mille motioned toward her daughter sitting across from her. "She's the youngest. When the time came, our regular doctor couldn't make it. He was too sick himself. If I remember, he had the flu bug or something. We had to send for another doctor who lived the next town over."

"How far away was that?" I asked.

"It was some fifteen miles away," Mille answered. "He had to come by horse and buggy. Not too many people living in the area had cars in those days." She looked at me and smiled. "Did you know that?"

"No, I guess I didn't."

"I didn't think so," Mille said as she continued on with her story. "I was sick in bed. I think I had some kind of toxic poisoning. Land sakes, I was sick," she exclaimed with raised eyebrows. "By the time the doctor arrived, I was having seizures. They tell me I was a sight for sore eyes. I was shaking so hard, the whole bed shook right along with me. I think that old doctor was worried about whether I would make it or not through the night. Although he didn't admit it, he sure looked scared." Mille took a sip of her champagne, smiled, and asked, "Are you sure you want to hear this?"

"I sure do."

"The doctor came in to where I was lying in bed. He had this tumbler full of a clear liquid. It had to be at least eight ounces." Mille picked up her water glass and showed me where eight ounces would come to. "He put the glass under his nose, smelled it, and then told me to drink it. Can you guess what it was?"

"The moonshine?"

"That's right." Mille giggled. "And it was ninety proof. My husband knew how to make it right," she exclaimed with obvious pride. "The doctor told me to drink that whole glass and as quickly as I could."

"My gosh." I smiled as I noticed Mille's daughter and son-in-law were doing their best to keep from laughing. They told me later that even though they had heard the story before, they cannot help being amused every time Mille tells it. "What happened?" I asked, trying to imagine drinking a whole glass of 90-proof moonshine.

"For one thing," Mille said with a chuckle, "I didn't have those seizures anymore." She chuckled again before going on. "I think I slept for the next two days. That old moonshine knocked me out cold. I don't remember anything. When I woke up, the doctor was still there. I don't know if he had been there all along, but he was sitting in the chair next to my bed. He looked so relieved that he jumped up from the chair and practically danced to the open window to take some deep breaths. That afternoon I gave birth to my ninth."

"What a story!" I exclaimed.

"Yes, sir," Mille agreed, "and when my baby was born, she was healthy." She gestured toward her daughter. "Why, you can see for yourself; this is the daughter who was born. It was that moonshine that did it."

"Mom," Mille's son-in-law said, "would you like another glass of champagne?" He had the bottle in his hand, ready to pour her a refill.

"No, thank you," Mille replied, waving the bottle away. "One drink is enough." She paused to finish the rest of the champagne in her glass. "Besides, it doesn't have much of a taste. It's too bubbly."

I thought to myself: *If Mille ever does become a resident at the nursing home I work at, I wonder what would happen when she got to know ninety-one-year-old Sadie.* You see, Sadie once confided in me that she knows all about *good moonshine*. And, oh yes, she still has the recipe.

Questions for Reflections

These questions are meant to be catalysts, to stimulate creative thinking about ways at providing quality, holistic care for the elderly. In some instances, the reflecting may lead to new (perhaps untraditional) ways of providing care. Not all questions may apply to your situation, but *all* situations will benefit from reflecting upon them. Whether your community is a long-term care facility, a new retirement home, or the old neighborhood, you can adapt them to fit your situation.

The Sailing Ship

1. Since death is a reality in our communities, it is important that we understand that the elderly think and talk about it a lot. With that in mind, discuss the following:
    a. The pros and cons of providing help to the elderly and their families in preplanning for death (e.g., offering seminars, workshops, etc.).
    b. If you are already doing some of 1a, what additional services could your community offer that would be beneficial? What are the needs of the elderly?

2. What assistance/support would be helpful to caretakers when they experience a death within their family or their circle of friends? (You may want to talk to caretakers who have already experienced a death. Ask them if they felt the support received from their workplace and community was helpful. Also ask, how could it be improved?)

Amazing Grace

1. Since few facilities have the luxury of having full-time chaplains as part of their staff, consider and discuss the following suggestions for promoting a better working relationship with

the spiritual leaders within the community:

    a. Facility could have an annual appreciation luncheon for them.

    b. Have facility resource people speak at their places of worship (to educate their people about such things as Alzheimer's, respite care, caring for aging parents, etc.)

    c. Ask ministers to come in for an open forum with staff at a facility. The purpose is to openly discuss a cooperative *and* mutually beneficial relationship.

2. If you could tap into existing groups who have a spiritual foundation and have been trained to provide care (e.g., Stephen Ministers, Befrienders, etc.), how would you use them?

3. Discuss the pros and cons of offering facilities in your community as a training ground for groups such as those in question 2.

Never a Wrong Number

1. This story speaks of a 94-year-old woman working in her garden. Consider having an outdoor garden (flowers, vegetables) for the elderly to help with and tend.

2. Both Beverly Mae's in the story have an attitude that exudes vitality for life. One of the definitions of vitality is "power, as of an institution to endure or survive." Keeping that definition in mind, evaluate your community's vitality by discussing the following:

    a. In what concrete and obvious ways do caretakers in your community exude the vitality of life in their jobs?

    b. In what ways could your community's vitality be nurtured?

Believing is Seeing

1. In the story, glasses that were lost were found. Within facilities, residents lose things. Some things, unfortunately, are stolen. So, if you are in a facility, consider the following:
    a. Does your facility offer basic training for on-the-job ethics? If not, how could you go about offering such training? Who would do it?
    b. Brainstorm and come up with a list of ethical behaviors for staff. (The definition of ethics is "a set of moral principals and values.")
    c. Have each department write a mission statement for practicing ethics within their area of work. (Be sure that all staff within that department are part of the process in developing the mission statement.)

2. Lost articles can also be a problem in an elderly person's home. What sorts of steps can be taken to ensure that important items are not lost or stolen? At what point should someone besides the elderly person begin to oversee financial matters?

He's Lying Again

1. It was said that Ernie was representative of the pets that residents had to leave behind when they entered the nursing home. For those not yet in a nursing home:
    a. Discuss the benefits (and drawbacks) of having a pet (such as a dog or cat).
    b. If dogs/cats are not an option, brainstorm what other animals could be pets.
    c. Discuss the pros and cons of having fish or birds as pets.

2. If you work in a facility, has it ever formally evaluated the benefits of having a facility pet? If not, how would you go

about doing so? Who authorizes such a study? You can look at question 1 for some of the other questions you might want to consider.

3. The puppet, Ernie, represented an untraditional approach in care giving. What kind of untraditional approaches would you like to use in your care giving?
    a. Who would you need to get approval from?
    b. Tough question: If you work in a facility, is it open to untraditional approaches to serving residents? If so, give examples how you are already doing so.

Moonshine Saved My Life

1. How do you feel about the elderly drinking alcoholic beverages? Do you consider alcoholism to be a concern in some cases?

2. If you are part of a facility, what is its policy on residents having alcoholic drinks (a glass of beer or wine)? If you have a policy against it, what is it based on? Who has the responsibility of reviewing such a policy?

3. What are the physical, emotional, and ethical issues for caretakers in dealing with a person who:
    a. Has AIDS (HIV) or another infectious disease.
    b. Has a past criminal record of committing violent crimes and is still prone to violence.

4. The number of elderly will be increasing in the near future and they will be from a different generation with different ideas about how life should be lived. Discuss the needs and demands of the next generation of elderly. How will this affect your community and your role in it?

5. Evaluate your preparedness in meeting those demands/needs in question 4.

6. What kind of changes will the long-term care industry face in the next five years?
    a. How will this impact the level of care facilities offer?
    b. If you are part of a facility, how will it affect *your* particular job?
    c. Will there be additional training needed for your job to face the future? If so, what is your facility doing to prepare you? What should it be doing?

Old age, to the unlearned, is winter; to the learned, it is harvest time.

— *Yiddish Proverb*

A Final Thought from the Author

It is my hope that you have seen these stories to be more than just sketches about elderly people who live in a nursing home, but rather as stories that are reminders of the common humanity we all share. Through these stories, it is also my hope that you now have a different perspective of life in a nursing home, but what is just as important is that you have been able to get a different perspective on life itself.

As you have read how the elderly experience life with all of its many twists and turns, I hope you have shared their laughter as well as their tears. Perhaps you also discovered that their *life values* such as freedom, the quest for independence, the right to live (and to die) with dignity, friendship, commitment, and caring for one another are values that are timeless and ageless.

Harold's philosophy to always aim for the bull's-eye challenges us to experience each day to its fullest. It also asks us to consider expanding our comfort zone; to attempt things in life that we never thought we could do.

Lester's question, *Do you ever visit the old and the sick?* is like a mirror; it is set before us so that we will take a reflective look at ourselves. His question calls us back to common values and reminds us what it means to care for one another.

Zelma's zest for life is an example of the enduring human spirit that has no age boundaries. Her positive approach to the challenges of life can serve as a role model for all of us.

All of the stories found within these pages are stories of people who have left us legacies to embrace. By embracing them, I believe our lives will be enriched.

Chaplain Chuck Tindell
14462 Upper Guthrie Ct.
Apple Valley, MN 55124